Biomarkers in Periodontal Health and Disease

Nurcan Buduneli

Biomarkers in Periodontal Health and Disease

Rationale, Benefits, and Future Directions

Springer

Nurcan Buduneli
Department of Periodontology
Faculty of Dentistry
Ege University
Izmir, Turkey

ISBN 978-3-030-37315-3 ISBN 978-3-030-37317-7 (eBook)
https://doi.org/10.1007/978-3-030-37317-7

This Springer imprint is published by the registered company Springer Nature Switzerland AG
The registered company address is: Gewerbestrasse 11, 6330 Cham, Switzerland

The supreme guide in life is science.
Do not be afraid of telling the truth.

Mustafa Kemal ATATÜRK

Dedicated to mom, who has always been the major encouraging power behind me; to dad, who had always believed in me
And to my dear daughter and son, who are my hope for the future

Preface

Periodontal diseases continue to be one of the most common chronic infectious and inflammatory diseases in the world. Pathogenic mechanisms acting in periodontal diseases contain two major arms: the microbial component and the host response. Knowledge on both aspects has been increasing tremendously during the last two decades. Indeed, the progress in knowledge and the available evidence have led European Federation of Periodontology and American Academy of Periodontology to combine power and build up a new classification system for periodontal diseases in 2017 after 18 years passed since the 1999 Classification.

Periodontology is one of the most glamorous fields of dentistry with dozens of exciting papers, which open up completely novel pathways of research. "The more we understand the scenario the more complex it becomes." This is quite true for periodontology. However, this complexity not only attracts even more scientists to work in this field but also stimulates building new bridges between various disciplines of dentistry and medicine to make the story clear.

Development of chair-side diagnostic tests for determining the presence or absence of periodontal disease and activity is still a challenge in periodontology. The use of biofluid samples such as gingival crevicular fluid, whole saliva, and serum as a means of evaluating host-derived products, as well as exogenous components has a great potential for diagnosis and monitorisation of periodontal diseases. Having more precise and early diagnostic tools may enable early intervention and help to develop individually tailored treatment modalities. We are not there, yet, but shall expect to arrive soon. The technological developments in laboratory methods and the closer collaboration with different branches of medicine bring great hope for the future. The spirit of positivity with "can do" and "will do" is definitely encouraging; however, it is clear that reliable biomarkers should base on strong evidence. I hope this monograph will help to fire more researchers working in the field of periodontology to get involved.

> Moonlight floods the whole sky from horizon to horizon
> How much it can fill your room depends on its windows.
> Mawlana Jalal-al-Din Rumi

İzmir, Anatolia
September 2019

Nurcan Buduneli

Acknowledgements

I am grateful to Dr. Burcu Kanmaz for kindly preparing all the illustrations and providing the photographs for this book.

Contents

1 Anatomy of Periodontal Tissues

Periodontal tissues comprise both soft and hard tissues and have unique features as such soft tissues are in close contact with the calcified tissues and there is always a biofilm around. The periodontium comprises four distinguished tissues gingiva, root cementum, periodontal ligament, and alveolar bone (Fig. 1.1). Altogether these tissues function as tooth supporting organ system and their severe destruction can lead tooth loss. The extracellular matrix of each periodontal tissue has fibrous and nonfibrous elements including collagens, elastin, fibronectin, laminin, osteopontin, bone sialoprotein, growth factors, proteoglycans, lipids, minerals, and water. The interactions between these components not only determine tissue health, but are also involved in tissue damage, repair, and regeneration. Tooth loss means loss of vital functions such as biting, chewing, speech, and aesthetics eventually causing decreased self-esteem as well as social problems. The primary aetiological factor for periodontal diseases is the microbial dental plaque or the oral biofilm. The microorganisms in the biofilm trigger host response and the activated inflammatory, immune cells cause tissue destruction. For successful periodontal treatment, it is imperative to clarify the disease causing agents together with the disease modifying factors. On the other hand, understanding the physiology of periodontal tissues is of utmost importance to develop protective strategies as well as new treatment modalities. Schroeder stated, "Insight into the architecture of (human) tissues is necessary to enable a creative mind to ask pertinent biological questions" (Schroeder 1997).

1.1 Healthy Periodontal Tissues

1.1.1 Gingiva

The gingiva is divided anatomically into marginal, attached, and interdental gingiva. The marginal or unattached gingiva is the terminal border of the gingiva surrounding the teeth in collar-like fashion. The free gingival groove is the border between the marginal and attached gingiva and visible in approximately half of the cases. The marginal gingiva is the soft tissue wall of the gingival sulcus, it is about 1 mm wide in normal and healthy periodontium and can be separated from the tooth surface with a periodontal probe.

The gingival sulcus is the shallow crevice around the tooth bounded by the tooth surface on one side and by the marginal gingiva on the other (Fig. 1.1). The clinical determination of the depth of gingival sulcus is an important diagnostic parameter. The clinically healthy gingiva has a sulcus depth of 1–3 mm.

The attached gingiva is continuous with the marginal gingiva and it is firm, resilient, and tightly bound to the underlying periosteum of alveolar bone. The width of attached gingiva is an important clinical parameter, extending

N. Buduneli, *Biomarkers in Periodontal Health and Disease*,
https://doi.org/10.1007/978-3-030-37317-7_1

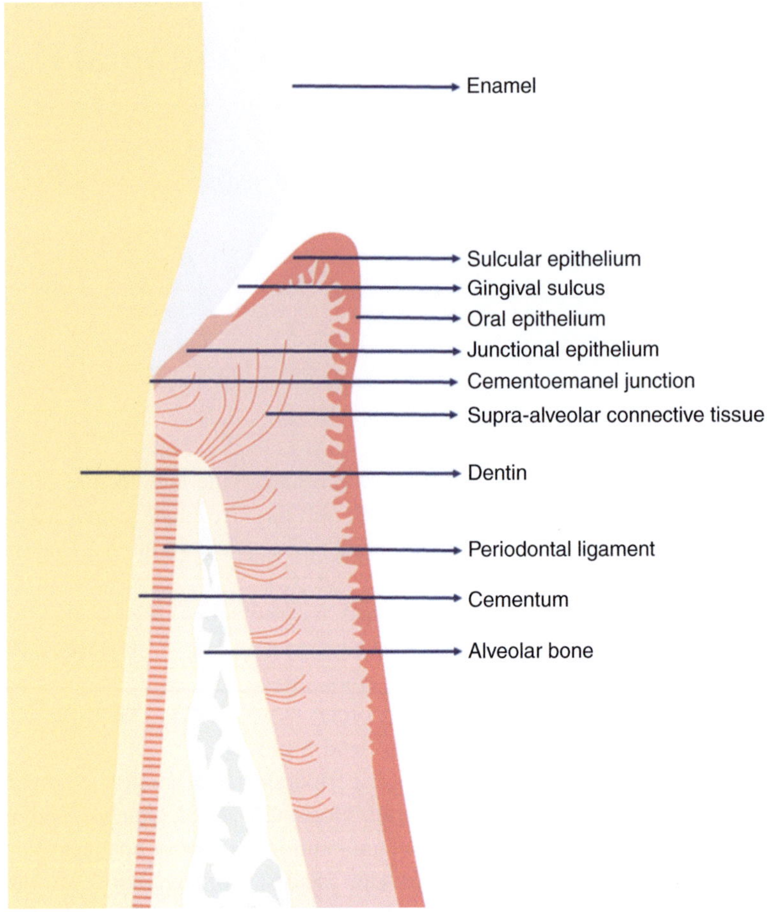

Fig. 1.1 Anatomy of the periodontal tissues

between the mucogingival junction and the projection on the external surface of the bottom of the gingival sulcus or periodontal pocket. The width of attached gingiva is greatest in the incisor region (3.5–4.5 mm in the maxilla and 3.3–3.9 mm in the mandible) and less in the posterior region, with the least width in the first premolar area (1.9 mm in the maxilla and 1.8 mm in the mandible).

Interdental gingiva normally occupies the gingival embrasure, which is the interproximal space beneath the area of tooth contact. Figure 1.2 shows an example of pristine healthy periodontium. It can be pyramidal or have a "col" shape. The shape of the interdental gingiva depends on the contact point between the two adjacent teeth. Presence or absence of gingival recession or hyperplasia directly affects the dimension and shape of the interdental gingiva.

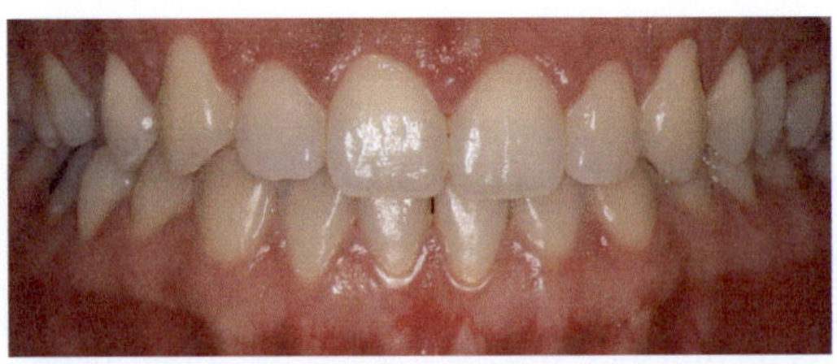

Fig. 1.2 Pristine healthy periodontal tissues

1.1.2 Dentogingival Junction

The dentogingival junction is the term to define the gingival portion facing the tooth surface and comprises both epithelial and connective tissue components. The epithelium has three components; gingival, sulcular, and junctional epithelium. Among these functional compartments, the junctional epithelium has very unique characteristics as it faces the calcified tooth surface and seals off periodontal tissues from the oral cavity. Therefore, it has to be intact in order to be able to protect deeper tissues from the microbiological, chemical, or physical inflammatory factors originating from the oral environment. The structural and functional uniqueness of the junctional epithelium makes it a very efficient barrier against periodontal pathogens and their virulence factors.

The junctional epithelium originates from the reduced enamel epithelium during the tooth eruption into the oral cavity. It is located around the cervical portion of the tooth as a collar at the level of cementoenamel junction (CEJ). It constitutes the base of the gingival sulcus. It is non-differentiated, stratified squamous epithelium and has a very high rate of cell turnover. It is thickest near the bottom of the gingival sulcus and ends with a few cells along the tooth surface. The epithelial attachment consists of a basal lamina-like structure that is adherent to the tooth surface that is a specialised extracellular matrix, which is rich in glycoconjugates. It also contains laminin 5, which mediates adhesion and migration of keratinocytes (Frank and Carter 2004).

The junctional epithelium cells contain fewer tonofilaments and desmosomes, and wider intercellular spaces compared to the gingival epithelium. These wide spaces contain polymorphonuclear leukocytes (PNL) and monocytes that originate from the subepithelial connective tissue and migrate into the gingival sulcus. Together with their enzymes these cells are the first line of defence against the microbial attacks from the oral biofilm. These cells can secrete molecules such as alpha (α)- and beta (β)-defensins, cathelicidin LL-37, interleukin (IL)-8, IL-1α, IL-1β, tumour necrosis factor-α, intercellular adhesion molecule-1 (ICAM-1), and lymphocyte function antigen-3 (LFA-3).

1.1.2.1 Connective Tissue

The connective tissue below the junctional epithelium differs structurally from that below the gingival epithelium. Even when the periodontal tissues are clinically healthy, there is always an infiltrate of inflammatory cells, mainly comprising PNLs. Also, T-lymphocytes continually migrate from the vessels in the connective tissue reaching out the gingival sulcus. The nature of the connective tissue beneath an epithelium has a determining role on the character of the epithelium. The subepithelial connective tissue provides instructive signals for the normal progression of the stratified squamous epithelia (Karring et al. 1971, 1975). The connective tissue immediately subjacent to the epithelium is rich in type I and type III collagen and also small proteoglycans decorin and biglycan. The basement membranes at the junctions of connective tissue with epithelium and cementum, the rete pegs, and the connective tissue around the blood vessels and nerves contain high amount of collagen type IV (Chavrier et al. 1984; Narayanan et al. 1985; Romanos et al. 1991).

1.1.3 Cementum

Cementum is the calcified avascular connective tissue that covers the roots of the teeth and is the periodontal tissue where the principal periodontal ligament fibres are attached. The ultrastructure of cementum is similar to that of bone and dentin (Selvig 1965). Basically, there are two types of cementum in regard with the presence or absence of cellular component and the origin of the collagen fibres of the extracellular matrix; acellular extrinsic fibre cementum and cellular intrinsic fibre cementum.

Acellular extrinsic fibre cementum, which is also called primary cementum or acellular cementum, exists on the cervical half to two thirds of the root. Sharpey's fibres are inserted in this portion of cementum, of which the overall degree of mineralisation is 45–60%.

Cellular intrinsic fibre cementum also called as the secondary cementum or cellular cementum is present along the apical third or half of the root and in furcation areas. It is produced as a repair tissue filling the resorptive defects and root fractures. Cementoblasts produce intrinsic collagen fibres and those cementoblasts entrapped in lacunae are called cementocytes. This type of cementum is less mineralised than the acellular extrinsic fibre cementum.

The cementum at and immediately subjacent to the CEJ is of particular clinical importance in root planing procedures. Moreover, this junction is the reference point for major clinical periodontal measurements. However, it does not exist in all teeth; in about 5–10% of cases cementum and enamel fails to meet leaving dentine exposed to the oral cavity.

In normal and healthy periodontium, cementum is placed in subgingival position and can become exposed to the oral cavity when there is gingival recession. In this case, organic substances, inorganic ions, and even bacteria can penetrate cementum. Indeed, bacterial penetration to cementum is common in periodontitis and non-surgical periodontal treatment aims to remove this infected cementum layer from the root surface.

Overall cementum contains about 50% mineral and 50% organic matrix. Its mineral content is about 65% by weight, which is a little more than that of bone. Approximately, 50% of the inorganic component of cementum is hydroxyapatite and 90% of the organic component is type I and III collagens (Birkedal-Hansen et al. 1977). Type III and type XII collagens are also found in high concentrations. There are trace amounts of other collagens, including type V, VI, and XIV. Moreover, there are non-collagenous matrix proteins, which are also found in alveolar bone (Bosshardt 2005). Among these there are bone sialoprotein, dentin sialoprotein, fibronectin, osteocalcin, osteonectin, osteopontin, tenascin, proteoglycans, proteolipids, and numerous growth factors such as insulin-like growth factor (IGF). Osteocalcin is a marker for maturation of osteoblasts, odontoblasts, and cementoblasts.

1.1.3.1 Molecular Factors that Regulate Cementogenesis

Bone morphogenetic proteins (BMP): These proteins are the members of the transforming growth factor-β (TGF-β) superfamily. Their exact functions have not been clarified but it is known that BMP-2, -4, and -7 promote the differentiation of preosteoblasts and putative cementoblast precursor cells.

Enzymes like alkaline phosphatase, matrix metalloproteinases, growth factors like TGF-β, IGF, and platelet-derived growth factor (PDGF), and proteoglycans also seem to have regulatory functions on cementoblast differentiation and activity.

1.1.4 Periodontal Ligament

Periodontal ligament is the soft, specialised connective tissue between the root cementum and alveolar bone. It communicates with the marrow spaces through vascular channels in the bone. Its width varies between 0.15 and 0.38 mm and its thinnest part is located around the middle third of the root length. Its thickness progressively decreases with age. Due to its resilience, periodontal ligament has unique functions such as acting as a shock absorber against the physiological and even traumatic forces coming towards the teeth. Moreover, it has sensory receptors necessary for the proper positioning of the jaws during mastication. It is also unique with its cell reservoir for tissue homeostasis and repair/regeneration.

Fibroblasts are the principal cells of the periodontal ligament and they are characterised by rapid turnover of the collagen content in the extracellular matrix. There are also epithelial cells in the periodontal ligament that are remnants of Malassez. Their function is unclear but it has been suggested that they may be involved in periodontal repair/regeneration. Moreover, there are undifferentiated mesenchymal cells in the periodontal ligament. During periodontal wound healing, the periodontal ligament cells contribute not only for its own repair but also for that of alveolar bone and cementum (Beertsen et al. 1997; Karring et al. 1993).

Collagen is a protein composed of different amino acids, the most important of which are glycine, proline, hydroxyproline, and hydroxylysine (Carneireo and Fava de Moraes 1965). Collagen is synthesised by fibroblasts, chondroblasts, osteoblasts, odontoblasts, and other cells. The predominant collagens of the periodontal ligament are type I, III, and XII. The collagen fibrils arranged in definite and distinct fibre bundles are termed as principal fibres. The embedded portions of the collagen fibres are called Sharpey's fibres. There are also elastic fibres in the periodontal ligament and they are oxytalan in nature. These fibres run more or less vertically from the cementum surface and form a three dimensional network that surrounds the root and terminates in the apical complex of arteries, veins, and lymphatics. These elastic fibres can expand in response to tensional forces. There are also non-collagenous matrix proteins in the periodontal ligament and these include alkaline phosphatase, proteoglycans, and glycoproteins such as tenascin and fibronectin. Tenascin is present in attachment zones along cementum and bone (Lukinmaa et al. 1991). Fibronectin and vitronectin are found in collagen fibrils.

Cellular component of periodontal ligament is mainly formed by connective tissue cells, epithelial rest cells, immune system cells, and cells associated with neurovascular elements (Berkovitz and Shore 1982).

Periodontal ligament also has a ground substance filling the spaces between the cells and the fibres. The major components of this ground substance are glycosaminoglycans and glycoproteins. Main glycosaminoglycans are hyaluronic acid and proteoglycans, whereas the main glycoproteins are fibronectin and laminin. The water content of periodontal ligament is high reaching about 70%.

The functions of periodontal ligament can be divided into three major groups; (1) physical functions, (2) formative and remodelling functions, and (3) nutritional and sensory functions. Within the context of physical functions periodontal ligament provides a soft tissue barrier for the vessels and nerves to protect them from injury by mechanical forces. Periodontal ligament transfers the occlusal forces to the alveolar bone, attaches the teeth to the bone, and provides resistance towards the occlusal forces by shock absorption. Periodontal ligament also has a role in the maintenance of the gingival tissues in their proper relationship to the teeth.

Within the context of formative and remodelling function, the periodontal ligament cells participate in the formation and resorption of cementum and bone and in the repair of injuries.

Finally, within the context of nutritional and sensory functions, the periodontal ligament supplies nutrients to the cementum, bone, and also gingiva by way of blood vessels and provides lymphatic drainage. There are abundant sensory nerve fibres capable of transmitting tactile, pressure, and pain sensations by the trigeminal pathways.

Periodontal ligament can adapt to functional changes. In case the functional demand increases, the width of periodontal ligament can increase up to 50% and the fibre bundles also increase in thickness. On the opposite, if the functional demand decreases, the ligament becomes narrower and the number as well as the thickness of the fibre bundles also decreases.

1.1.5 Alveolar Bone

The alveolar bone is the portion of the jaws that contain the roots of the teeth. It forms when the tooth erupts to provide the osseous attachment to the forming periodontal ligament. Accordingly, it disappears gradually when the tooth is lost. According to the stage of development and microstructure, bone can be divided into different types such as primary (woven), secondary (lamellar), cancellous (trabecular), and compact (cortical) (Buck and Dumanian 2012). There are outer cortical plates at both sides of the alveol and the spongious/trabecular bone between them. The bone lining the socket is called as the bundle bone since it is the region of attachment for the periodontal ligament fibre bundles. The cortical plates consist of surface layers supported by Haversian systems. The trabecular or spongious bone also consists of bone disposed in lamellae, with Haversian systems.

The turnover of the alveolar bone is very rapid and following tooth extraction the edentulous part of the alveolar bone is resorbed in both horizontal and vertical directions. The factors that control homeostasis of the periodontal tissues still need to be better explained. If and when these mechanisms are fully understood, it may be possible to guide tissue healing after non-surgical or surgical periodontal treatment.

With a macro-scale; collagen fibres are aligned according to the mechanical and functional requirements of the tissue and with a nano-scale; cross-linked collagen matrices are embedded within a mineralised matrix (Bartold et al. 2019). Similar to the other periodontal tissues, the predominant organic component of the alveolar bone are type I and III collagens (Wang et al. 1980). There are also biologically active polypeptides such as bone sialoprotein and osteopontin (Chen et al. 1993). The major proteoglycans are rich in chondroitin sulphate (Bartold 1990; Waddington and Embery 1991).

The cellular component of alveolar bone includes osteoblasts that differentiate from pluripotent follicle cells. Then, there are osteocytes that are enclosed within spaces called lacunae. Osteoclasts are bone-resorbing cells that originate from haematopoietic tissue. Active osteoclasts possess an elaborately developed ruffled border from which the hydrolytic enzymes are released (Vaes 1988).

Alveolar bone has a number of functions; it provides mechanical support and protection, maintains the mineral homeostasis, haematopoiesis, and also has endocrine functions (Florencio-Silva et al. 2015).

1.2 Blood Supply of the Periodontium

The gingiva, periodontal ligament, and alveolar bone are rich in blood vessels, whereas the cementum is an avascular tissue. The gingiva receives its blood supply from the supraperiosteal blood vessels, vessels of the periodontal ligament, and also from the arterioles that emerge from the alveolar crest to the interdental septa. Subepithelial plexus is located immediately beneath the oral epithelium. The capillary loops reach into the oral epithelium. The dentogingival plexus is located beneath the junctional epithelium.

1.3 Lymphatic System of the Periodontium

The smallest lymph vessels, the lymph capillaries, form an extensive network in the connective tissue. The lymph is absorbed from the tissue fluid through the thin walls into the lymph capillaries. The lymph vessels are similar to veins as they are provided with valves. The periodontal tissues have connections with the submental, deep cervical, submandibular, and jugulodigastric lymph nodes.

1.4 Nerves of the Periodontium

The periodontium contains mechanoreceptors that record pain, touch, and pressure. In addition to these, the periodontal ligament also contains proprioreceptors that give information about the movements and positions. The small nerves of the periodontium follow almost the same course with the blood vessels. Gingival innervation is derived from fibres arising from nerves in the periodontal ligament as well as from the labial, buccal, and palatal nerves.

1.5 Stem Cells of the Periodontium

Stem cells in general originate from four sources: embryonic tissues, foetal tissues, postnatal tissues, and reprogrammed differentiated somatic cells that are termed “inducible pluripotent stem cells” (Lin et al. 2008). Mesenchymal stem cells (MSC) include cells derived from nearly all tissues in the human body and depending on their source these cells can differentiate into adipocytes, osteoblasts, chondrocytes, tenocytes, skeletal myocytes, and visceral stromal cells (Gronthos et al. 2003; Horwitz et al. 1999; Jiang et al. 2002).

References

Bartold PM. A biochemical and immunohistochemical study of the proteoglycans of alveolar bone. J Dent Res. 1990;69:7–19.

Bartold P, Gronthos S, Haynes D, Ivanovski S. Mesenchymal stem cells and biologic factors leading to bone formation. J Clin Periodontol. 2019;46(Suppl.21):12–32.

Beertsen W, Van Den Bos T, Everst V. Continuous growth of acellular extrinsic fiber cementum: a review. Acta Med Dent Helv. 1997;2:103–15.

Berkovitz BKB, Shore RC. Cells of the periodontal ligament. In: Berkovitz BKB, Moxham BJ, Newman HE, editors. The periodontal ligament in health and disease. London: Pergamon Press; 1982.

Birkedal-Hansen H, Butler WT, Taylor RE. Proteins of the periodontium. Characterization of the insoluble collagens of bovine dental cementum. Calcif Tiss Res. 1977;23:39–44.

Bosshardt DD. Are cementoblasts a subpopulation of osteoblasts or a unique phenotype? J Dent Res. 2005;84:390–406.

Buck DW, Dumanian GA. Bone biology and physiology: part I. the fundamentals. Plastic Reconst Surg. 2012;129:1314–20.

Carneiro J, Fava de Moraes F. Radioautographic visualisation of collagen metabolism in the periodontal tissues of the mouse. Arch Oral Biol. 1965;10:833–46.

Chavrier C, Couble ML, Magloire H, Grimaud JA. Connective tissue organisation of healthy human gingiva. Ultrastructural localization of collagen types I-III-IV. J Periodontal Res. 1984;19:221–9.

Chen J, McCulloch CA, Sodek J. Bone sialoprotein in developing porcine dental tissues: cellular expression and comparison of tissue localization with osteopontin and osteonectin. Arch Oral Biol. 1993;38:241–9.

Florencio-Silva R, Sasso GR, Sasso-Cerri E, Simoes MJ, Cerri PS. Biology of bone tissue: structure, function, and factors that influence bone cells. Biomed Res Int. 2015;2015:421746.

Frank DE, Carter WG. Laminin 5 deposition regulates keratinocyte polarisation and persistent migration. J Cell Sci. 2004;117:1351–63.

Gronthos S, Chen S, Wang CY, Robey PG, Shi S. Telomerase accelerates of osteoclastogenesis of bone marrow stromal stem cells by upregulation of CBFA1, osterix, and osteoclacin. J Bone Miner Res. 2003;18:716–22.

Horwitz EM, Prockop DJ, Fitzpatrick LA, Koo WW, Gordon PL, Neel M, et al. Transplantability and therapeutic effects of bone marrow-derived mesenchymal cells in children with osteogenesis imperfect. Nature Med. 1999;5:309–13.

Jiang Y, Jahagirdar BN, Reinhardt RL, Schwartz RE, Keene CD, Ortiz-Gonzales XR, et al. Pluripotency of mesenchymal stem cells derived from adult marrow. Nature. 2002;418:41–9.

Karring T, Ostergaard E, Loe H. Conservation of tissue specificity after heterotopic transplantation of gingiva and alveolar mucosa. J Periodontal Res. 1971;6:282–93.

Karring T, Lang NP, Loe H. The role of gingival connective tissue in determining epithelial differentiation. J Periodontal Res. 1975;10:1–11.

Karring T, Nyman S, Gottlow J, Laurell L. Development of the biological concept of guided tissue regeneration-animal and human studies. Periodontol 2000. 1993;1:26–35.

Lin NH, Gronthos S, Bartold PM. Stem cells and periodontal regeneration. Aust Dent J. 2008;53:108–21.

Lukinmaa PL, Mackie EJ, Thesleff I. Immunohistochemical localization of the matrix glycoproteins-tenascin and the ED-sequence-containing form of cellular fibronectin in human permanent teeth and periodontal ligament. J Dent Res. 1991;70:19–26.

Narayanan AS, Clagett JA, Page RC. Effect of inflammation on the distribution of collagen types I, III, IV, and V and type I trimer and fibronection in human gingivae. J Dent Res. 1985;64:1111–6.

Romanos G, Schröter-Kermani C, Hinz N, Bernimoulin J-P. Immunohistochemical distribution of the collagen types IV, V, VI, and glycoprotein laminin in the healthy rat, marmoset (Callithrix jacchus) and human gingivae. Matrix. 1991;11:125–32.

Schroeder HE. Biological structure of the normal and diseased periodontium-preface. Periodontol. 1997;13:17.

Selvig KA. The fine structure of human cementum. Acta Odontol Scand. 1965;23:423–41.

Vaes G. Cellular biology and biochemical mechanism of bone resorption. Clin Orthop. 1988;231:239–71.

Waddington RJ, Embery G. Structural characterization of human alveolar bone proteoglycans. Arch Oral Biol. 1991;36:859–66.

Wang HM, Nanda V, Rao LG, Melcher AH, Heersche JN, Sodek J. Specific immunohistochemical localization of type III collagen in porcine periodontal tissues using the peroxidase-antiperoxidase method. J Histochem Cytochem. 1980;28:1215–23.

Nature of Periodontal Diseases

2

The clinical manifestations of periodontal disease are the result of very complex interactions between the microorganisms in the oral cavity that form the microbial dental plaque and the host response towards the microorganisms and their virulence factors. It is clear that periodontal diseases are multifactorial and apart from the microbial factors that trigger the host immune response, the genetic background of the host, the systemic health, environmental conditions like smoking and psychological stress, and various medications used for the treatment of systemic diseases can all affect the clinical outcome.

2.1 Inflammation

Inflammation is the central pathologic feature of periodontal disease and the microbial dental plaque is the major aetiological factor. The immune and inflammatory responses are critical to the pathogenesis of periodontitis. The initial response to the oral biofilm is a local inflammatory reaction that activates the innate immune system (Graves and Cochran 2003; Garlet et al. 2006). In case, this innate inflammatory response is not controlled by feedback mechanisms or the host cells are hyper reactive, an array of various cytokines, enzymes, and other mediators are released leading to connective tissue destruction and bone resorption. In case of periodontitis, there are also alterations in bone metabolism. Two critical factors are now regarded as determining whether bone loss will occur and these are; the concentration of inflammatory mediators present in gingival tissue to be sufficient to activate pathways leading to bone resorption and the other is the penetration of the inflammatory mediators to gingival tissue to reach a critical distance to alveolar bone (Graves and Cochran 2003). Hence, bacteria are necessary for disease initiation, but they are not sufficient to cause tissue destruction (Page 1998). It is becoming quite clear that the mechanisms for soft tissue destruction are not completely same with those for calcified tissue destruction. There is a continuous remodelling in soft and hard tissues of periodontium, but the mechanisms of tissue renewal in health differ from the pathogenic mechanism acting in disease. Possibly, not only the main actors, but also the reactions or interactions may differ in this context.

Periodontitis is described as a multifactorial, irreversible, and cumulative condition, initiated and propagated by bacteria and host factors (Kinane 2001). It continues to be the most common cause of tooth loss worldwide. The immune and inflammatory responses are orchestrated by a number of host-related factors, either intrinsic or acquired (Taubman et al. 2005). Under normal physiological conditions there is a balance between bone formation and bone resorption. In other words, osteoblastic and osteoclastic functions are balanced. Bone

N. Buduneli, *Biomarkers in Periodontal Health and Disease*,
https://doi.org/10.1007/978-3-030-37317-7_2

homeostasis is maintained as long as this balance is preserved. When the structural integrity and/or calcium metabolism is altered, this balance is lost towards either increased bone formation or bone resorption. There are examples of systemic diseases/conditions such as rheumatoid arthritis and osteoporosis and also local diseases such as periodontitis.

A principal feature of inflammatory periodontitis is enhanced osteoclast activity without a corresponding increase in bone formation. Osteoclasts are the principal cells responsible for bone resorption in periodontitis that are multinucleated cells deriving from the monocyte-macrophage lineage (Boyle et al. 2003; Lerner 2000; Rubin and Greenfield 2005). Both experimental studies in animal models and human studies indicated that multinucleated osteoclasts resorb alveolar bone. A variety of cytokines play role in formation of cytokines (Fig. 2.1). The relationship between the immune system and bone metabolism has been termed "osteoimmunology" and this is a rapidly progressing field of research (Arron and Choi 2000). Clarifying the mechanism of osteoimmunology seems to be promising for the development of new prevention and treatment modalities for bone loss in periodontitis. As clearly explained recently by Bosshardt (2018) transformation of the junctional epithelium to the pocket epithelium is

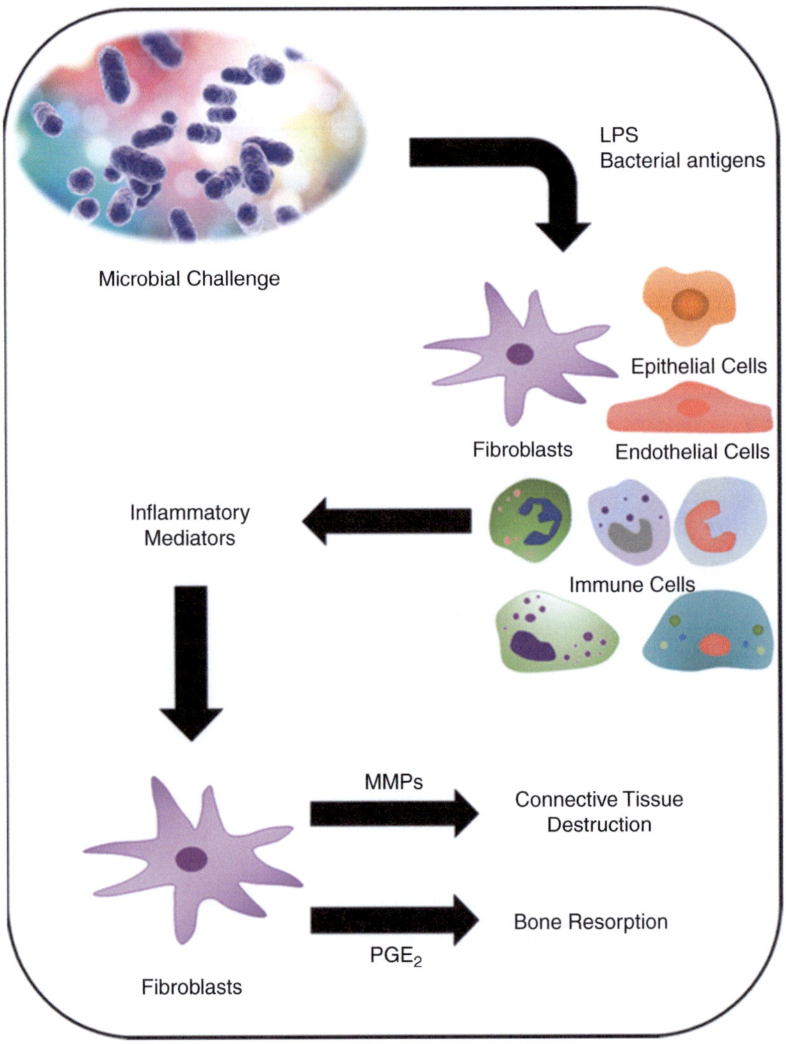

Fig. 2.1 Inflammatory mechanisms in alveolar bone resorption

critical in the onset of periodontitis. The timepoint of this transformation is regarded as pivotal for the pocket formation. Bosshardt (2018) and Nibali (2018) suggested that the influence of virulence factors might be important in the breakdown of the junctional epithelium leading to pocket formation. The biofilm's influences on the junctional epithelium destabilising it by thinning and/or ulceration that results in further subgingival spread of the bacteria are quite clear.

A variety of molecular, cellular, and immunohistochemical events take place during the progression of gingivitis to periodontitis (Kurgan and Kantarci 2018). Histologically, there are four phases in this progression; initial lesion, early lesion, established lesion, and advanced lesion (Page and Schroeder 1976). The initial lesion is the response of resident leukocytes and endothelial cells to the dental biofilm.

At this stage, there is no clinical sign of inflammation and this lesion can only be detected by histological investigation. Upon stimulus from bacteria and their virulence factors, junctional epithelium cells produce cytokines, neutrons produce neuropeptides, vascular changes comprising vasodilatation and increase in permeability occur. Neutrophils leave the vessels and start migrating towards the centre of inflammation. In the early lesion, the number of neutrophils is increased in the inflamed connective tissue and macrophages, lymphocytes, plasma cells, and mast cells start to appear in the lesion. The junctional epithelium proliferates forming rete pegs. Early clinical signs of inflammation such as redness and bleeding become visible. Flow of the gingival crevicular fluid increases. The established lesion is considered as the stage of transition from innate response to acquired immune response, where there are dominating numbers of T-lymphocytes, macrophages, B-lymphocytes, and plasma cells. There is an increase in blood flow and collagenolytic activity. Collagen production by fibroblasts is also increased. Clinically, this stage is recognised as moderate to severe gingivitis with easily detectable changes in the colour, contour, consistence changes in gingiva. The final stage of advanced lesion defines the transition from gingivitis to periodontitis. There is irreversible tissue destruction with attachment loss, bone resorption, and connective tissue degradation. Bone loss becomes clinically detectable. This model indicated that most of the tissue destruction in periodontitis is caused by host responses to the biofilm microorganisms.

The old concept that untreated gingivitis would inevitably progress to periodontitis has been refuted by the data from longitudinal epidemiologic studies (Ismail et al. 1990; Listgarten et al. 1985; Löe et al. 1978, 1986, 1992). Gingivitis always precedes periodontitis but not all cases of gingivitis progresses to periodontitis. On the contrary, only a fraction of untreated sites with gingivitis progressed to periodontitis during the observation period. Later studies revealed that untreated periodontitis often progresses in people who are not on regular maintenance recall programs (Axelsson and Lindhe 1978, 1981). It then became clear that there was no way to determine either the risk or the presence of periodontal disease activity at a single visit (Hancock 1981).

Today, it is accepted that anything that increases susceptibility to infections, or alters their destructive course, may serve as a risk factor for periodontitis. Risk factors may be modifiable or nonmodifiable. However, currently, there is no fully validated formal risk-assessment method for estimating the risk of progression, or the recurrence of periodontitis (Garcia et al. 2009; Loos et al. 2005).

2.2 Pathogen Microorganisms

Since the first reports showing the role of bacteria in periodontal disease onset, there have been significant changes in the context of microbiological aetiology of periodontal diseases (Guerini 1909, 1981). First, there was the "non-specific plaque hypothesis" stating that the extent and severity of periodontal disease are proportional to the amount of plaque accumulating on teeth surfaces. This hypothesis was refuted, as there were cases with significant amounts of plaque but no clear sign or symptom of periodontal disease. Then came the "specific plaque hypothesis" claiming that some certain bacteria rather than the bulk of plaque play a major role in the onset and progression of periodontal disease Löesche (Löesche 1976). So, the content of plaque became much more important than its amount. Later on, research revealed that more or less same bacteria species were present in the healthy and diseased individuals as well as the healthy and diseased sites. Hence, the specific plaque hypothesis was also refuted. The third plaque hypothesis; "ecological plaque hypothesis" included the environmental factors and the host into the frame together with the bacteria in the plaque; the start and progression of periodontal disease is dependent on the presence of pathogenic bacteria in a susceptible host and environmental factors, such as smoking, uncontrolled diabetes, genetic background, etc., increase the severity of periodontal tissue destruction (Marsh 2003). Today, this multifactorial scenario continues to be the most appropriate to explain the pathogenic mechanisms of periodontitis (Fig. 2.2).

The exact mechanisms of periodontal tissue breakdown are not clearly understood but disease onset and progression invariably involves a disruption of the homeostasis or balance between the resident microbiota and the host (Listgarten 1986; Darveau 2010). Periodontal homeostasis can be disrupted by a variety of host- or microbe-related factors. Congenital or acquired host immunodeficiencies, immunoregulatory defects associated with mutations or polymorphisms, old age, systemic diseases such as diabetes, obesity, environmental factors (smoking, diet, and stress), epigenetic modifications in response to environmental changes, and the presence of keystone pathogens can transform a symbiotic microbiota into a dysbiotic one (Stabholz et al. 2010; Zhou et al. 2011; Eskan et al. 2012; Hajishengallis et al. 2012; Laine et al. 2012; Divaris et al. 2013; Lindroth and Park 2013; Hajishengallis 2014). The dysbiosis is not dependent so much on the particular microbial roster but rather on the specific gene combinations or collective viru-

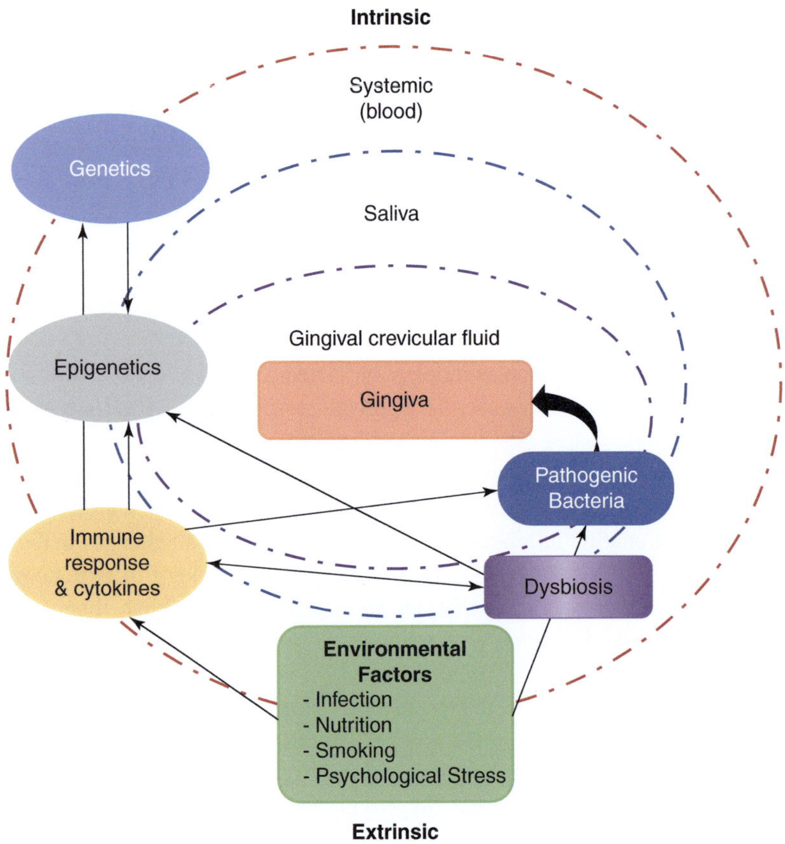

Fig. 2.2 Multifactorial pathogenic mechanisms acting in periodontitis

lence activity within the microbial community (Hajishengallis and Lamont 2012). Accordingly, a recent study employed gene expression profiling to characterise patient-matched healthy and disease-associated periodontal microbiotas (Jorth et al. 2014). It was reported that disease-associated microbial communities exhibit highly conserved metabolic gene expression profiles, despite high interpatient variability in microbial composition.

Sigmund Socransky understood that periodontal infections were caused by organised communities of bacteria in which some microorganisms were more important than others from an etiological point of view and he proposed a set of criteria to be used while determining if a microorganism is likely to be an etiological agent in periodontal diseases (Socransky 1979). These criteria were patterned after Koch's postulates and included the following: association with disease; elimination or suppression of the organism results in disease remission; host response (i.e., detection of adaptive immune responses to the organism); demonstration that the organism is pathogenic in an experimental animal; and—the organism should possess an array of virulence factors that can be linked to the pathogenesis of periodontal inflammation. "Socransky Criteria" were used to generate lists of periodontopathogens in the World Workshop held in 1996 (Genco et al. 1996). The workshop participants agreed that there is a strong evidence for pathogen status of *Porphyromonas gingivalis, Tannerella forsythia,* and *Aggregatibacter actinomycetemcomitans*. Moderate evidence exists to support the pathogenic role of *Campylobacter rectus, Eubacterium nodatum, Prevotella intermedia/nigrescens, Parvimonas micra, Treponema denticola,* and the *Streptococcus milleri*. During the following years studies were published focusing on one or two of these putative pathogens. However, this attitude could never reflect the truth, as it has never been accepted that periodontal diseases occur as a monoinfection. Indeed, the complex metabolic interactions between different species of bacteria have a greater role in the tissue destruction rather than the virulence factors of one or two specific bacteria (Fig. 2.3). Periodontal diseases are polymicrobial infections (Socransky and Haffajee 2005). Indeed, the

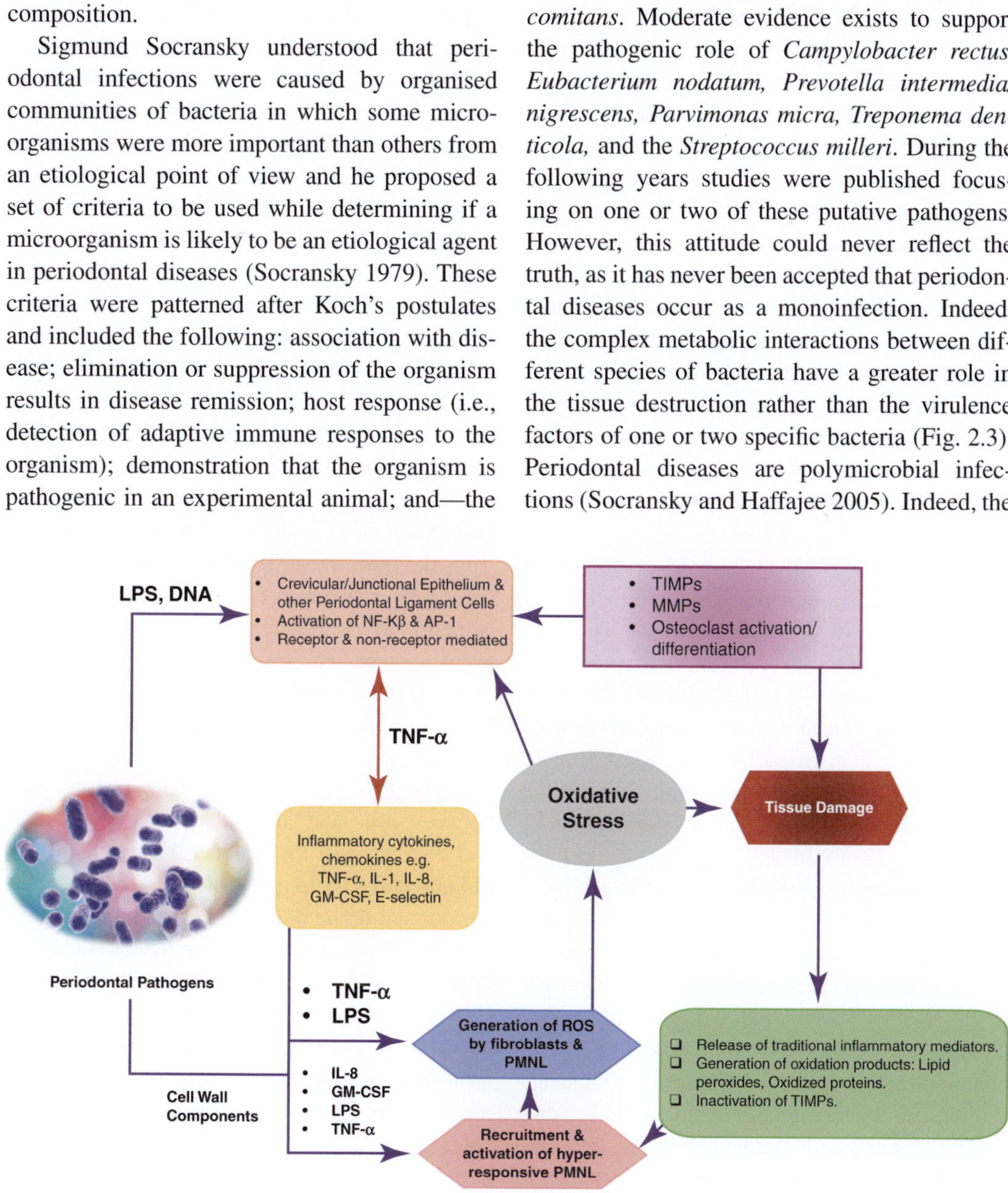

Fig. 2.3 Complex interactions between pathogen microorganisms and host response in the aetiopathogenesis of periodontitis

polymicrobial nature of periodontitis explains why routine microbial testing, as part of the treatment planning for periodontitis appears to have limited clinical value (Shaddox and Walker 2009). Accordingly, a systematic review failed to report high-level evidence supporting the diagnostic value of microbial testing in the management of periodontitis (Listgarten and Loomer 2003). The microbial component of periodontal diseases is usually composed of flora bacteria that are more or less present in many individuals in the society and sites in a mouth. These bacteria are a normal part of the health-associated oral microbiota and only become pathogens when there is a major disturbance in the host-microbe homeostasis (Armitage 2013). Therefore, the pathogens are considered as opportunistic and endogenous. This issue decreases the utility of microbial testing for diagnostic and/or monitoring purposes. Such tests may be beneficial in selected cases, where the response to periodontal treatment fails to be satisfactory or as expected.

2.3 Immune Response

Innate and adaptive host immune responses to the microorganisms in the oral biofilm lead to the destruction of periodontal tissues. The host immune response can contribute to protective and/or destructive effects in periodontal diseases. As part of the innate response, neutrophils pass from the highly vascularised gingival tissue to the gingival crevice and form a wall between the host tissue and the dental plaque biofilm (Tonetti et al. 1998). Approximately, 30,000 polymorphonuclear neutrophils (PMNs) transit through periodontal tissue every minute. The architecture and permeability of the junctional epithelium permit this migration of cells. Adhesion molecules such as E-selectin, intercellular adhesion molecules (ICAMs), cytokines such as interleukin (IL)-8, and other molecules such as human β-defensins, soluble and membrane-bound CD14, and lipopolysaccharide-binding protein (LBP) all affect immune cell functions against dental biofilm bacteria (Tonetti et al. 1998; Jin and Darveau 2001; Jin et al. 2004; Ren et al. 2004).

Oral epithelial cells have tight intercellular junctions that form a mechanical barrier to the entry of bacteria and their toxins. Lipopolysaccharide (LPS) is the cell-wall component of gram-negative bacteria that triggers host response. Dendritic cells present antigens such as LPS to other immune cells for antibody production. Recognition of innate immune signals by dendritic cells relies on a limited number of pathogen-related receptors. Toll-like receptors (TLRs) are among these proteins that regulate apoptosis, inflammation, and immune responses (Anderson 2000). This family of receptors are expressed on lymphocytes, osteoclast precursors, macrophages, osteoblasts, epithelial cells, and stromal cells (Hayashi et al. 2003). Clinically healthy gingival tissue also expresses a variety of TLRs possibly acting in the inflammatory response of periodontium (Darveau 2010). Eleven different TLR molecules have been identified in human periodontal tissues so far (Liu et al. 2010). The binding of TLRs with pathogen-associated molecules leads to the production of cytokines, chemokines, and antimicrobial peptides. TLR-2 and TLR-4 are the dominant ones in periodontal tissues and they can differentiate microorganisms from the host. TLRs are capable of recognising pathogens, can regulate a host innate immune response to periodontopathic bacteria and can serve as a bridge between innate and adaptive immune responses (Song et al. 2017). They are likely to play a central role in the initiation and progression of periodontitis.

In healthy periodontium, there is a balance between pro- and anti-inflammatory cytokines and disruption of this balance in favour of pro-inflammatory cytokines may contribute to the periodontal tissue damage. Certain bacteria such as *P. gingivalis* are suspected to have a role in the disruption of this balance and tissue homeostasis. However, no single oral bacteria species seems to be the only disruptor. Rather than this, as bacterial numbers increase, the proteases found in the red complex bacteria (*Porphyromonas gingivalis, Tannerella forsythia,* and *Aggregatibacter actinomycetemcomitans*) may further compromise innate defence by inactivating potentially protective host responses (Darveau 2010).

2.4 Osteoclastic Bone Resorption

Enhanced osteoclast activity is a basic component of bone loss in inflammatory periodontitis (Cochran 2008, Gruber 2019). Particular attention focuses on receptor activator of NF-kappaB ligand (RANKL), a member of the tumour necrosis factor ligand family, because this molecule plays a key role in osteoclastogenesis (Yasuda et al. 1998; Kong et al. 1999). Osteoblasts are the major cells expressing RANKL, but at sites of inflammation other cells such as fibroblasts, T-lymphocytes, B-lymphocytes also express this ligand (Teitelbaum 2007). Parathyroid hormone, vitamin D3, and cytokines like interleukin (IL)-1, IL-11 also have regulatory functions on RANKL expression (Lacey et al. 1998; Matsuzaki et al. 1998; Hofbauer and Heufelder 2001; Caetoano-Lopes et al. 2009). Osteoprotegerin (OPG) is the natural inhibitor of RANK, it acts as a decoy, competes with RANK to bind RANKL. In case the concentration of OPG is high enough, it binds RANKL inhibiting the binding of RANK and RANKL. Human periodontal ligament cells, gingival fibroblasts, and epithelial cells can produce OPG and inflammatory cytokines such as transforming growth factor-β (TGF-β) can modulate its expression (Sakata et al. 1999; Kanzaki et al. 2002).

It was reported that the osteoblasts express more RANKL than do the osteoclasts (Fumoto et al. 2014). Hence, different than the previous thoughts, osteoblasts are now considered to have a significant role in osteoclastic bone resorption. Osteoclasts can bind to mineralised bone surface, but there is always a non-mineralised layer of bone called "osteoid" covering bone surfaces and the first step in bone resorption is the degradation of this osteoid layer. Collagenolytic enzymes of the flat and elongated cells at the top of the osteoid degrade this non-mineralised layer thereby enhancing osteoclastic bone resorption (Chambers and Fuller 1985).

Macrophage colony stimulating factor (M-CSF) produced mainly by osteoblasts or bone marrow stromal cells plays a significant role in osteoclast development and activation leading to alveolar bone loss (Bartold et al. 2010). Proliferation and survival of preosteoclasts and also mature osteoclasts are promoted by M-CSF (Chambers 2000).

2.5 Network of Cytokines and Chemokines

Cytokines and chemotactic cytokines (chemokines) transmit the messages between various cells and the immune response is regulated by these interactions. Cytokines are low-molecular-weight proteins involved in the initiation as well as progression of inflammation. Secretion of pro-inflammatory cytokines from a variety of cells usually starts with the activation of nuclear factor kappaB (NFkB) (Hanada and Yoshimura 2002) (Fig. 2.3). Resident cells like epithelial cells, fibroblasts and blood cells like neutrophils and macrophages secrete cytokines during acute and early chronic phases of inflammation, whereas lymphocytes secrete cytokines during established and advanced phases of inflammation. Interleukin (IL)-1 and IL-6 are those cytokines first discovered within the context of periodontal inflammation. They are characteristically related with inflammatory cell migration and osteoclastogenesis (Fonseca et al. 2009). Tumour necrosis factor-alpha (TNF-α) is a multi-potent cytokine functioning from cell migration to tissue destruction. TNF-α upregulates secretion of IL-1beta and IL-6 and it is also correlated with extracellular matrix degradation and bone resorption via promoting MMPs and RANKL (Fig. 2.4).

Pro-inflammatory cytokines such as IL-1β, IL-6, IL-11, IL-17, and TNF-α can induce osteoclastogenesis by increasing the expression of RANKL and decreasing OPG production by osteoblasts/stromal cells (Nakashima et al. 2000). When there is abundant OPG expression, but reduced RANKL, the net ratio of RANKL/OPG becomes smaller and the outcome is likely to be excessive formation of bone. On the contrary, when there is a relative decrease in OPG concentration, or an increase in that of RANKL, or both happening at the same time, then there is an excessive bone resorption due to the net

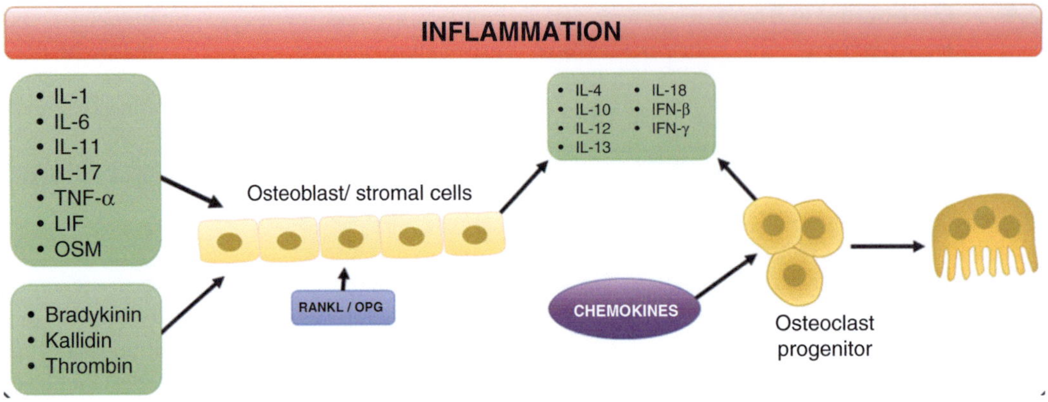

Fig. 2.4 Cytokines and chemokines in bone resorption

increase in the RANKL/OPG ratio. IL-17 is of particular importance due to its increasing effect on RANKL expression and concomitantly decreasing effect on OPG expression in osteoblastic cells in vitro and in vivo, thereby enhancing osteoclast formation and bone erosion in a mouse model of arthritis (Lubberts et al. 2003). Just the opposite, anti-inflammatory cytokines such as IL-13 and interferon (IFN)-γ, have lowering effect on RANKL expression and/or increasing effect on that of OPG, eventually inhibiting osteoclastogenesis (Nakashima et al. 2000). IFN-γ also plays a major role in B-cell maturation. It is present at high levels in periodontal lesions and associated with progression of periodontitis (Dutzan et al. 2009).

IL-4 is another important anti-inflammatory cytokine acting in proliferation of T-cells and regulating B-cell secretions. It inhibits the production of MMPs and RANKL, at the same time induces upregulation of tissue inhibitors of MMPs (TIMPs) and OPG. It is regarded as a protective cytokine in the pathogenesis of periodontal diseases. It also induces the production of another anti-inflammatory cytokine IL-10. This cytokine plays a direct protective role in tissue destruction by downregulating both MMPs and RANKL. Transforming growth factor-beta (TGF-β) regulates cell growth, differentiation, and matrix production and also is a potent immunosuppressive factor that downregulates the transcription of pro-inflammatory cytokines such as IL-1β and TNF-α. In active periodontal lesions, the levels of TGF-β negatively correlate with those of RANKL (Dutzan et al. 2009).

Chemokines are small proteins that play significant roles in chemotactic migration of cells to the site of infection. Endothelial cells, epithelial cells, stromal cells, as well as leukocytes can secrete chemokines. They are grouped as homeostatic or inflammatory (Moser et al. 2004). They are essential signals for the trafficking of osteoblast and osteoclast precursors, potentially modulating also bone homeostasis. Chemokines can effectively contribute to bone remodelling by driving osteoblast migration and activation.

2.6 Lipid Mediators of Inflammation

Prostaglandins (PGs) are derived from the hydrolysis of cell membrane phospholipids. Arachidonic acid is metabolised by either lipoxygenases or cyclooxygenases (COXs). PGE2 is a potent stimulator of alveolar bone resorption. At high concentrations, PGE2 decreases the levels of IgG, but at low concentrations it has the potential to increase IgG (Fig. 2.5).

Offenbacher et al. (2007) proposed a "biologic systems model" as a critical framework with which the components of the periodontal disease may be seen. This model incorporates all components that contribute to the final clinical phenotype, which is the clinical presentation of the disease. Later on, the authors hypothesised that there are different biologic factors underlying periodontal disease in different individuals (Offenbacher et al. 2008).

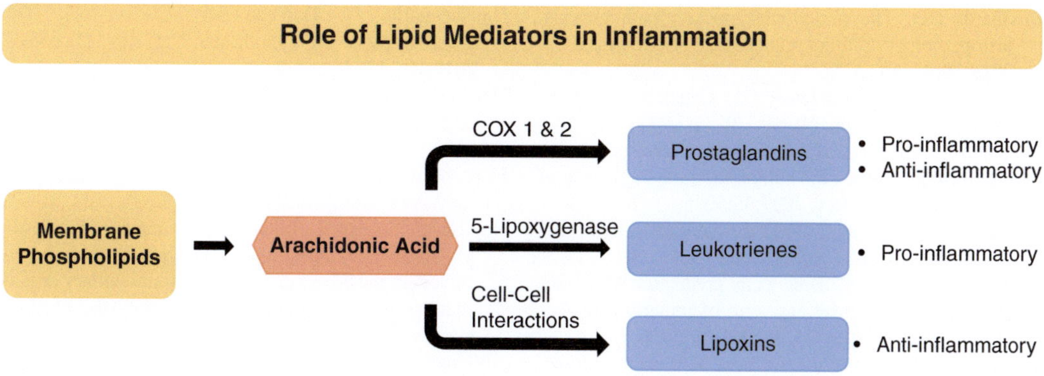

Fig. 2.5 Lipid mediators acting in bone resorption

In the healthy state, there is a balance between bone resorption and bone formation (Boyle et al. 2003). Excessive bone formation can be observed in certain inflammatory conditions such osteopetrosis and excessive bone resorption can be observed in chronic diseases such as osteoporosis and periodontitis (Lerner 2006; Saidenberg-Kermanach et al. 2004). Very recently, Lerner et al. (2019) outlined the complex events taking place in the osteoclastic bone resorption. First, secreted osteoclast factors such as bone morphogenetic protein (BMP)-6 act on osteoblasts. Secondly, membrane-bound osteoclast-derived factors act on osteoblasts. Thirdly, matrix-derived factors such as BMP-2,-4,-5,-6,-7,-9, insulin-like growth factor (IGF)-1 act on osteoblasts. Fourthly, factors such as TGF-β act directly on osteoclasts. Then, there are factors such as IGF-1 acting indirectly on osteoclasts by regulating RANKL/OPG ratio. Later on, osteocyte-derived factors act on osteoblasts, and finally, osteocyte-derived factors act on osteoclasts. This scenario clearly indicates that osteoclastic bone resorption comprises very complex mechanisms and not only osteoclasts but also osteoblasts play critical roles in osteoclastic bone resorption.

2.7 Conclusion

As a conclusion, the pathogenic mechanism acting in periodontal tissue destruction is clearly complex and multifactorial. The clinical phenotype seems to be the ultimate outcome of the complex interactions between the biologic phenotype in terms of cellular and molecular host responses and surrogate biomarkers, genetic and epigenetic composition including race, age, and gender, and finally individual risk factors such as smoking, diabetes, obesity, and the individual composition of the dental biofilm. The genotype is a determining factor for predisposition as well as for the phenotype. Understanding the biological background of the phenotypes of periodontal diseases may eventually help to establish prognosis and develop individually tailored treatment modalities for active and maintenance phases of periodontal therapy.

References

Anderson KV. Toll signalling pathways in the innate immune response. Curr Opin Immunol. 2000;12:13–9.

Armitage GC. Learned and unlearned concepts in periodontal diagnostics: a 50-year perspective. Periodontol 2000. 2013;62:20–36.

Arron JR, Choi Y. Bone versus immune system. Nature. 2000;408:535–6.

Axelsson P, Lindhe J. Effect of controlled oral hygiene procedures on caries and periodontal disease in adults. J Clin Periodontol. 1978;5:133–51.

Axelsson P, Lindhe J. Effect of controlled oral hygiene procedures on caries and periodontal disease in adults. Results after 6 years. J Clin Periodontol. 1981;8:239–48.

Bartold PM, Cantley MD, Haynes DR. Mechanisms and control of pathologic bone loss in periodontitis. Periodontol. 2010;53:55–69.

Bosshardt DD. The periodontal pocket: pathogenesis, histopathology and consequences. Periodontol 2000. 2018;76:43–50.

Boyle WJ, Simonet WS, Lacey DL. Osteoclast differentiation and activation. Nature. 2003;423:337–42.

Caetoano-Lopes J, Canhao H, Fonseca JE. Osteoimmunology—the hidden immune regulation of bone. Autoimmun Rev. 2009;8:250–5.

Chambers TJ. Regulation of the differentiation and function of osteoclasts. J Pathol. 2000;192:4–13.

Chambers TJ, Fuller K. Bone cells predispose bone surfaces to resorption by exposure of mineral to osteoclastic contact. J Cell Sci. 1985;76:155–65.

Cochran DL. Inflammation and bone loss in periodontal disease. J Periodontol. 2008;79:1569–76.

Darveau RP. Periodontitis: a polymicrobial disruption of host homeostasis. Nat Rev Microbiol. 2010;8:481–90.

Divaris K, Monda KL, North KE, et al. Exploring the genetic basis of chronic periodontitis: a genome-wide association study. Hum Mol Genet. 2013;22:2312–24.

Dutzan N, Vernal R, Hernandez M, Dezerega A, Rivera O, Silva N, Aguillon JC, Puente J, Pozo P, Gamonal J. Levels of interferon-gamma and transcription factor T-bet in progressive periodontal lesions in patients with chronic periodontitis. J Periodontol. 2009;80:290–6.

Eskan MA, Jotwani R, Abe T, et al. The leukocyte integrin antagonist Del-1 inhibits IL-17-mediated inflammatory bone loss. Nat Immunol. 2012;13:465–73.

Fonseca JE, Santos MJ, Canhao H, Choy E. Interleukin-6 as a key player in systemic inflammation and joint destruction. Autoimmun Rev. 2009;8:538–42.

Fumoto T, Takeshita S, Ito M, Ikeda K. Physiological functions of osteoblast lineage and T cell-derived RANKL in bone homeostasis. J Bone Miner Res. 2014;29:830–42.

Garcia RI, Nunn ME, Dietrich T. Risk calculation and periodontal outcomes. Periodontol. 2009;50:65–77.

Garlet GP, Cardoso CR, Silva TA, et al. Cytokine pattern determines the progression of experimental periodontal disease induced by *Actinobacillus actinomycetemcomitans* through the modulation of MMPs, RANKL, and their physiological inhibitors. Oral Microbiol Immunol. 2006;21:12–20.

Genco R, Kornman K, Williams R, et al. Consensus report. Periodontal disease: pathogenesis and microbial factors. Ann Periodontol. 1996;1:926–32.

Graves DT, Cochran D. The contribution of interleukin-1 and tumour necrosis factor to periodontal tissue destruction. J Periodontol. 2003;74:391–401.

Gruber R. Osteoimmunology: inflammatory osteolysis and regeneration of the alveolar bone. J Clin Periodontol. 2019;46(Suppl. 21):52–69.

Guerini V. History of dentistry. Philadelphia: Lea & Febiger; 1909.

Guerini V. History of dentistry. Odontostomatol Proodos. 1981;35:198–204.

Hajishengallis G. Aging and its impact on innate immunity and inflammation: implications for periodontitis. J Oral Biosci. 2014;56:30–7.

Hajishengallis G, Lamont RJ. Beyond the red complex and into more complexity: the polymicrobial synergy and dysbiosis (PSD) model of periodontal disease etiology. Mol Oral Microbiol. 2012;27:409–19.

Hajishengallis G, Darveau RP, Curtis MA. The keystone-pathogen hypothesis. Nat Rev Microbiol. 2012;10:717–25.

Hanada T, Yoshimura A. Regulation of cytokine signalling and inflammation. Cytokine Growth Factor Rev. 2002;13:413–21.

Hancock EB. Determination of periodontal disease activity. J Periodontol. 1981;52:492–9.

Hayashi S, Yamada T, Tsuneto M, Yamane T, Takahashi M, Shultz LD, Yamazaki H. Distinct osteoclast precursors in the bone marrow and extramedullary organs characterised by responsiveness to toll-like receptor ligands and TNF-alpha. J Immunol. 2003;171:5130–9.

Hofbauer LC, Heufelder AE. Role of receptor activator of nuclear factor-kappaB ligand and osteoprotegerin in bone cell biology. J Mol Med. 2001;79:243–53.

Ismail AI, Morrison EC, Burt BA, Caffesse RG, Kavanagh MT. Natural history of periodontal disease in adults: findings from the Tecumseh periodontal disease study 1959-87. J Dent Res. 1990;69:430–5.

Jin L, Darveau RP. Soluble CD14 levels in gingival crevicular fluid of subjects with untreated adult periodontitis. J Periodontol. 2001;72:634–40.

Jin L, Ren L, Leung WK, Darveau RP. The in vivo expression of membrane-bound CD14 in periodontal health and disease. J Periodontol. 2004;75:578–85.

Jorth P, Turner KH, Gumus P, Nizam N, Buduneli N, Whiteley M. Metatranscriptomics of the human oral microbiome during health and disease. MBio. 2014;5:e01012–4.

Kanzaki H, Chiba M, Shimizu Y, Mitanı H. Periodontal ligament cells under mechanical stress induce osteoclastogenesis by receptor activator of nuclear factor kappaB ligand up-regulation via prostaglandin E2 synthesis. J Bone Miner Res. 2002;17:210–20.

Kinane DF. Causation and pathogenesis of periodontal disease. Periodontol 2000. 2001;25:8–20.

Kong YY, Feige U, Sarosi I, et al. Activated T cells regulate bone loss and joint destruction in adjuvant arthritis through osteoprotegerin ligand. Nature. 1999;402:304–9.

Kurgan S, Kantarci A. Molecular basis for immunohistochemical and inflammatory changes during progression of gingivitis to periodontitis. Periodontol 2000. 2018;76:51–67.

Lacey DL, Timms E, Tan HL, Kelley MJ, Dunstan CR, Burgess T, et al. Osteoprotegerin ligand is a cytokine that regulates osteoclast differentiation and activation. Cell. 1998;93:165–76.

Laine ML, Crielaard W, Loos BG. Genetic susceptibility to periodontitis. Periodontol 2000. 2012;58:37–68.

Lerner UH. Osteoclast formation and resorption. Matrix Biol. 2000;19:107–20.

Lerner UH. Inflammation-induced bone remodelling in periodontal disease and the influence of post-menopausal osteoporosis. J Dent Res. 2006;85:596–607.

Lerner UH, Kindstedt E, Lundberg P. The critical interplay between bone resorbing and bone forming cells. J Clin Periodontol. 2019;21:33–51.

Lindroth AM, Park YJ. Epigenetic biomarkers: a step forward for understanding periodontitis. J Periodontal Implant Sci. 2013;43:111–20.

Listgarten MA. Pathogenesis of periodontitis. J Clin Periodontol. 1986;13:418–25.

Listgarten MA, Loomer PM. Microbial identification in the management of periodontal diseases. A systematic review. Ann Periodontol. 2003;8:182–92.

Listgarten MA, Schiffer CC, Laster I. 3-year longitudinal study of the periodontal status of an adult population with gingivitis. J Clin Periodontol. 1985;12:225–38.

Liu YC, Lerner UH, Teng YT. Cytokine responses against periodontal infection: protective and destructive roles. Periodontol 2000. 2010;52:163–206.

Löe H, Anerud A, Boysen H, Smith M. The natural history of periodontal disease in man: the rate of periodontal destruction before 40 year of age. J Periodontol. 1978;49:607–20.

Löe H, Anerud A, Boysen H, Morrison E. Natural history of periodontal disease in man: rapid, moderate and no loss of attachment in Sri Lankan laborers 14 to 46 years of age. J Clin Periodontol. 1986;13:431–40.

Löe H, Anerud A, Boysen H. The natural history of periodontal disease in man: prevalence, severity, and extent of gingival recession. J Periodontol. 1992;63:489–95.

Löesche WJ. Chemotherapy of dental plaque infections. Oral Sci Rev. 1976;9:65–107.

Loos BG, John RP, Laine ML. Identification of genetic risk factors for periodontitis and possible mechanisms of action. J Clin Periodontol. 2005;32(Suppl. 6):159–1679.

Lubberts E, Bersselaar L, Oppers-Walgreen B, et al. IL-17 promotes bone erosion in murine collagen-induced arthritis through loss of the receptor activator of NF-kappa B ligand/osteoprotegerin balance. J Immunol. 2003;170:2655–62.

Marsh PD. Are dental diseases examples of ecological catastrophes? Microbiology. 2003;149:279–94.

Matsuzaki K, Udagawa N, Takahashi N, Yamaguchi K, Yasuda H, Shima N, et al. Osteoclast differentiation factor (ODF) induces osteoclast-like cell formation in human peripheral blood mononuclear cell cultures. Biochem Biophys Res Commun. 1998;246:199–204.

Moser B, Wolf M, Walz A, Loetscher P. Chemokines: multiple levels of leukocyte migration control. Trends Immunol. 2004;25:75–84.

Nakashima T, Kobayashi Y, Yamasaki S, et al. Protein expression and functional difference of membrane-bound and soluble receptor activator of NF-kappaB ligand: modulation of the expression by osteotropic factors and cytokines. Biochem Biophys Res Commun. 2000;275:768–75.

Nibali L. Development of the gingival sulcus at the time of tooth eruption and the influence of genetic factors. Periodontol 2000. 2018;76:35–42.

Offenbacher S, Barros SP, Singer RE, Moss K, Williams RC, Beck JD. Periodontal disease at the biofilm-gingival interface. J Periodontol. 2007;78:1911–25.

Offenbacher S, Barros SP, Beck JD. Rethinking periodontal inflammation. J Periodontol. 2008;79:1577–84.

Page RC. The pathobiology of periodontal diseases may affect systemic diseases: inversion of a paradigm. Ann Periodontol. 1998;3:108–20.

Page RC, Schroeder HE. Pathogenesis of inflammatory periodontal disease. A summary of current work. Lab Invest. 1976;34:235–49.

Ren L, Jin L, Leung WK. Local expression of lipopolysaccharide-binding protein in human gingival tissues. J Periodontal Res. 2004;39:242–8.

Rubin J, Greenfield E. Osteoclast origin and differentiation. In: Bronner F, Frach-Carson MC, Rubin J, editors. Topics in bone biology-bone Resorption, vol. 2. London: Springer; 2005. p. 1–23.

Saidenberg-Kermanach N, Cohen-Solal M, Bessis N, De Vernejoul MC, Boisser MC. Role for osteoprotegerin in rheumatoid inflammation. Joint Bone Spine. 2004;71:9–13.

Sakata M, Shiba H, Komatsuzawa H, Fujita T, Ohta K, Sugai M, Suginaka H, Kurihara H. Expression of osteoprotegerin (osteoclastogenesis inhibitory factor) in cultures of human dental mesenchymal cells and epithelial cells. J Bone Miner Res. 1999;14:1486–92.

Shaddox LM, Walker C. Microbial testing in periodontics: value, limitations and future directions. Periodontol 2000. 2009;50:25–38.

Socransky SS. Criteria for the infectious agents in dental caries and periodontal disease. J Clin Periodontol. 1979;6(Extra issue):16–21.

Socransky SS, Haffajee AD. Periodontal microbial ecology. Periodontol 2000. 2005;38:135–87.

Song B, Zhang YL, Chen LJ, Zhou T, Huang WK, Zhou X, Shao LQ. The role of toll-like receptors in periodontitis. Oral Dis. 2017;23:168–80.

Stabholz A, Soskolne WA, Shapira L. Genetic and environmental risk factors for chronic periodontitis and aggressive periodontitis. Periodontol. 2010;53:138–53.

Taubman MA, Valvende P, Han X, Kawai T. Immune response: the key to bone resorption in periodontal disease. J Periodontol. 2005;76:2033–41.

Teitelbaum SL. Osteoclasts: what do they do and how do they do it? Am J Pathol. 2007;170:427–35.

Tonetti MS, Imboden MA, Lang NP. Neutrophil migration into the gingival sulcus is associated with transepithelial gradients of interleukin-8 and ICAM-1. J Periodontol. 1998;69:1139–47.

Yasuda H, Shima N, Nakagawa N, et al. Osteoclast differentiation factor is a ligand for osteoprotegerin/osteoclastogenesis-inhibitory factor and is identical to TRANCE/RANKL. Proc Natl Acad Sci USA. 1998;95:3597–602.

Zhou Q, Leeman SE, Amar A. Signalling mechanisms in the restoration of impaired immune function due to diet-induced obesity. Proc Natl Acad Sci USA. 2011;108:2867–72.

3 Conventional Diagnosis of Periodontal Diseases and the 2017 Classification System

Diagnosis is defined as the act of identifying a disease from its signs and symptoms. On the other hand, classification is defined as the act or method of distribution into groups. Diagnosis of a disease can also be regarded as the "best guess" of the clinician about the health problem of the particular patient.

Diseases of the tooth supporting structures have been mentioned in ancient medical works. In 1723, Fauchard used a specific name for the first time in history to define periodontal disease as "scurvy of the gums" (Gold 1985). Since then, various names related to etiological factors, pathological changes, or clinical manifestations have been used by researchers. Gottlieb is considered as the first author, who clearly distinguished various forms of periodontal disease and he classified periodontal disease into four types (Gottlieb 1920, 1923, 1928). At about the same time, McCall and Box (1925) introduced the term "periodontitis" to define the inflammatory periodontal disease, which affect gingiva, bone, and periodontal ligament. Since then, various classifications have been suggested. Page and Schroeder (1981) defined periodontitis as an inflammatory disease of the periodontium characterised by the presence of periodontal pocketing and active bone resorption with acute inflammation. At least four distinct periodontitis types were proposed; prepubertal periodontitis, juvenile periodontitis, rapidly progressive periodontitis, adult periodontitis, and acute necrotising ulcerative gingivitis-periodontitis (ANUG/ANUP). In their system, age of onset was the major determining factor.

3.1 1989 Classification of Periodontal Diseases

In 1989, World Workshop in Clinical Periodontics was held and the following classification was recommended (AAP 1989):

1. Adult periodontitis.
2. Early onset periodontitis.
   (a) Prepubertal periodontitis.
      - Generalised.
      - Localised.
   (b) Juvenile periodontitis
      - Generalised.
      - Localised.
   (c) Rapidly progressive periodontitis.
3. Periodontitis associated with systemic diseases.
4. Necrotising ulcerative periodontitis.
5. Refractory periodontitis.

This 1989 classification system had major drawbacks such as extensive overlap between the different diagnostic categories, the need for assumptions concerning previous disease progression, the necessity for detailed information on the quality of previous periodontal treatments

N. Buduneli, *Biomarkers in Periodontal Health and Disease*,
https://doi.org/10.1007/978-3-030-37317-7_3

provided, and the apparent lack of a consistent basis for classification (van der Velden, 2017).

3.2 1999 Classification of Periodontal Disease

Ten years later, a new classification system was built at the International Workshop for a Classification of Periodontal Diseases and Conditions (Armitage 1999). The discriminative role of age of disease onset was diminished in this new system and new terms were proposed that do directly refer neither the age of onset nor the responsiveness to the periodontal treatment.

1. Gingival diseases.
   (a) Dental plaque-induced gingival diseases.
   (b) Non-plaque-induced gingival lesions.
2. Chronic periodontitis (mild, moderate, severe).
   (a) Localised.
   (b) Generalised.
3. Aggressive periodontitis (mild, moderate, severe).
   (a) Localised.
   (b) Generalised.
4. Periodontitis as manifestation of systemic diseases.
   (a) Associated with haematological disorders.
   (b) Associated with genetic disorders.
   (c) Not otherwise specified.
5. Necrotising periodontal diseases.
   (a) Necrotising ulcerative gingivitis.
   (b) Necrotising ulcerative periodontitis.
6. Abscesses of periodontium.
   (a) Gingival abscess.
   (b) Periodontal abscess.
   (c) Pericoronal abscess.
7. Periodontitis associated with endodontic lesions.
   (a) Combined periodontic-endodontic lesions.
8. Developmental or acquired deformities and conditions.
   (a) Localised tooth-related factors that modify or predispose to plaque-induced gingival diseases/periodontitis.
   (b) Mucogingival deformities and conditions around teeth.
   (c) Mucogingival deformities and conditions on edentulous ridges.
   (d) Occlusal trauma.

The 1999 classification system mainly relied on the progression rate of periodontitis and chronic periodontitis indicated a slow progression of alveolar bone loss, whereas aggressive periodontitis defined a rapidly progressing form. This system was used worldwide for 18 years and many clinicians as well as researchers had difficulties in applying this system. The 1999 classification resulted in no conceptual changes (Armitage 1999, 2002). The major problem was faced in discrimination of chronic and aggressive periodontitis forms. This difficulty was preventing data combination coming from different research centres.

3.3 2017 Classification of Periodontal Diseases

A new classification system has been developed for periodontal diseases in 2017 World Workshop in order to accommodate advances from biological and clinical research performed since the 1999 Classification. This joint workshop of European Federation of Periodontology (EFP) and American Academy of Periodontology (AAP) aimed to develop a system that would be simple to use for not only the periodontists but also for the general practitioners. There is no more distinction between chronic and aggressive periodontitis since there was unconvincing biological evidence that these two were distinct entities. Only the classical localised juvenile (aggressive) periodontitis remains as a separate phenotype. According to the 2017 classification, the three types of periodontitis are as follows (Papapanou et al. 2018):

- Necrotising periodontitis.
- Periodontitis.
- Periodontitis as a manifestation of systemic disease.

The new classification system confirms that once a periodontitis patient, always a periodontitis patient, due to the fact that periodontitis may recur or progress at any time if periodontal maintenance is not optimal and risk factors are not eliminated or controlled. When a patient is diagnosed to have periodontitis, then staging and grading should be performed. The staging of periodontitis reflects the disease severity at presentation, which is also associated with the complexity of overall patient management (Table 3.1). Hence, the goals of staging are: firstly to classify severity and extent of an individual based on currently measurable extent of destroyed and damaged tissue attributable to periodontitis and secondly to assess specific factors that may determine complexity of controlling current disease and managing long-term function and aesthetics of the patient's dentition. The grading on the other hand is designed to reflect the patient's susceptibility to periodontitis because historical disease experience at a given age essentially accommodates all risk determinants for bone loss (Table 3.2). Hence, the goals of the grading can be outlined as follows: firstly to estimate future risk of periodontitis progression and responsiveness to standard therapeutic principles, to guide intensity of therapy and monitoring and secondly to estimate potential health impact of periodontitis on systemic disease and the reverse to guide systemic monitoring and co-therapy with medical colleagues (Tonetti et al. 2018).

The initial stage should be determined using clinical attachment loss (CAL); if not available, then radiographic bone loss (RBL) should be used. Information on tooth loss that can be attributed primarily to periodontitis—if available—may modify stage definition. This is the case even in the absence of complexity factors. Complexity factors may shift the stage to a higher level, for example, furcation II or III would shift to either stage III or IV irrespective of CAL. The distinction between stage III and stage IV is primarily based on complexity factors. For example,

Table 3.1 Classification of periodontitis based on stages defined by severity (according to the level of interdental clinical attachment loss, radiographic bone loss and tooth loss), complexity and extent and distribution

Periodontitis stage		Stage I	Stage II	Stage III	Stage IV
Severity	Interdental CAL at site of greatest loss	1–2 mm	3–4 mm	≥5 mm	≥5 mm
	Radiographic boneloss	Coronal third (<15%)	Coronal third (15%–33%)	Extending to mid-third of root and beyond	Extending to mid-third of root and beyond
	Tooth loss	No tooth loss due to periodontitis		Tooth loss due to periodontitis of ≤4 teeth	Tooth loss due to periodontitis of ≥5 teeth
Complexity	Local	Maximum probing depth ≤4 mm Mostly horizontal bone loss	Maximum probing depth ≤5 mm Mostly horizontal bone loss	In addition to stage II complexity: Probing depth ≥6 mm Vertical bone loss ≥3 mm Furcation involvement class II or III Moderate ridge defect	In addition to stage III complexity: Need for complex rehabilitation due to: Masticatory dysfunction secondary occlusal trauma (tooth mobility degree ≥2) Severe ridge defect Bite collapse, drifting, flaring Less than 20 remaining teeth (10 opposing pairs)
Extent and distribution	Add to stage as descriptor	For each stage, describe extent as localised (<30% of teeth involved), generalised, or molar/incisor pattern			

Table 3.2 Classification of periodontitis based on grades that reflect biologic features of the disease including evidence of, or risk for, rapid progression, anticipated treatment response, and effects on systemic health

Periodontitis grade			Grade A: slow rate of progression	Grade B: moderate rate of progression	Grade C: rapid rate of progression
Primary criteria	Direct evidence of progression	Longitudinal data (radiographicbone loss or CAL)	Evidence of no loss over 5 years	<2 mm over 5 years	≥2 mm over 5 years
	Indirect evidence of progression	% bone loss/age	<0.25	0.25–1.0	>1.0
		Case phenotype	Heavy biofilm deposits with low levels of destruction	Destruction commensurate with biofilm deposits	Destruction exceeds expectation given biofilm deposits; specific clinical patterns suggestive of periods of rapid progression and/or early onset disease (e.g., molar/incisor pattern; lack of expected response to standard bacterial control therapies)
Grade modifiers	Risk factors	Smoking	Non-smoker	Smoker <10 cigarettes/day	Smoker ≥10 cigarettes/day
		Diabetes	Normoglycaemic/ no diagnosis of diabetes	HbA1c <7.0% in patients with diabetes	HbA1c ≥7.0% in patients with diabetes

a high level of tooth mobility and/or posterior bite collapse would indicate a stage IV diagnosis. For any given case only some, not all, complexity factors may be present, however, in general it only takes one complexity factor to shift the diagnosis to a higher stage. It should be emphasised that these case definitions are guidelines that should be applied using sound clinical judgment to arrive at the most appropriate clinical diagnosis. For post-treatment patients, CAL and RBL are still the primary stage determinants. If a stage-shifting complexity factor(s) is eliminated by treatment, the stage should not retrogress to a lower stage since the original stage complexity factor should always be considered in maintenance phase management.

The proposed grading system included biomarkers but, due to the lack of strong and globalised evidence, this was not possible. However, the new classification is a live system and updates will be possible by a task force to accommodate future advances in biomarker research.

Grade should be used as an indicator of the rate of periodontitis progression. The primary criteria are either direct or indirect evidence of progression. Whenever available, direct evidence is used; in its absence indirect estimation is made using bone loss as a function of age at the most affected tooth or case presentation (radiographic bone loss expressed as percentage of root length divided by the age of the subject, RBL/age). Clinicians should initially assume grade B disease and seek specific evidence to shift towards grade A or C, if available. Once grade is established based on evidence of progression, it can be modified based on the presence of risk factors. CAL = clinical attachment loss; HbA1c = glycated haemoglobin A1c; RBL = radiographic bone loss.

From the clinical point of view, it is essential to determine whether the categorisation is clinically meaningful, and whether it enables the clinician to better customise treatment and improve treatment outcomes. Indeed, the demand for individually tailored treatment protocols is increasing not only from the health care providers' but also from the patients' perspective. A very recent study compared the periodontitis patients' classifications between the 1999 and 2018 systems (Graetz et al. 2019). The researchers followed

251 periodontitis patients for a mean follow-up duration of 21 years and concluded that the 2019 classification well reflected patients' characteristics, disease severity/extent/progression, and tooth loss.

Periodontal diseases are roughly divided into two categories as gingivitis and periodontitis (Fig. 3.1). Gingivitis defines inflammation in the gingiva and the clinical signs are restricted to swelling, redness, bleeding on probing, and contour changes of the gingival tissue. All these changes are reversible and gingivitis heals perfectly well after the etiological factors are removed. Periodontitis, on the other hand, is characterised by the destruction of connective tissue, loss of periodontal attachment, and resorption of alveolar bone. The tissue destruction observed in periodontitis is irreversible.

3.4 Medical and Dental History

Obtaining a detailed patient history is the first step and then clinical periodontal measurements are the basic and mandatory tools for periodontal diagnosis. Patient's medical and dental history should be recorded by asking simple and clear questions. The importance of medical history should be explained to the patient as some people often omit information that they cannot relate to their dental problems. A two-way relationship has been reported or at least suspected between periodontal diseases and some systemic diseases or conditions. A variety of systemic diseases, conditions, or behavioural factors may have a role in the onset and progression of periodontal diseases. On the other hand, severe periodontitis may adversely affect the course of some endocrine and cardiovascular diseases. Therefore, presence of diabetes, cardiovascular diseases, allergy, and infectious diseases should be systematically questioned. The major complaint of the patient should be noted. Current usage of medications, tobacco products, and home care routine should be asked. Heavy smokers are regarded as having a high risk for disease progression, and therefore, smokers should be identified during periodontal examination and counselled to modify this behavioural risk factor (Buduneli and Kinane 2011) (Fig. 3.2). Family medical history and oral health of family members and the presence or frequency of environmental smoking should also be questioned.

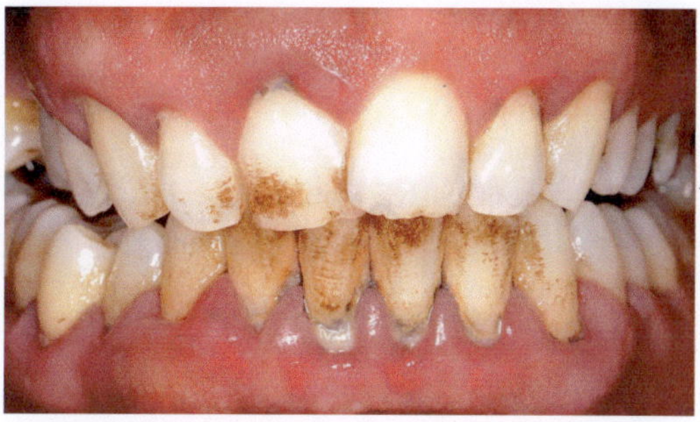

Fig. 3.2 Typical findings in a smoker; staining on the teeth, relatively less clinical signs of gingival inflammation

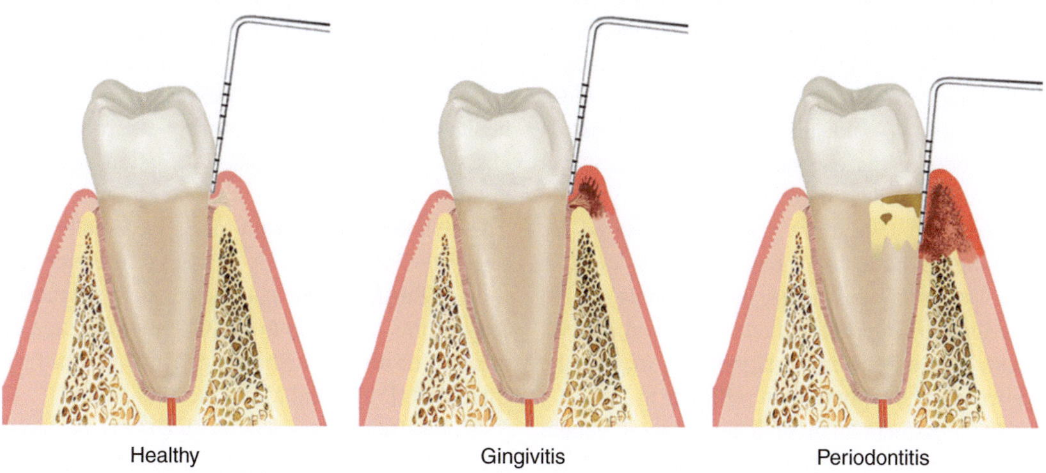

Fig. 3.1 Illustration of clinical diagnosis of healthy periodontium, gingivitis, and periodontitis

Key points in patient interview:

- Source of referral (dentist or physician).
- Chief complaint (usually there is none).
- Symptoms (bleeding, tooth migration, abscess).
- Medical and dental history (previous and present diseases, treatments).

3.5 Clinical Periodontal Parameters

A full-mouth comprehensive periodontal evaluation follows the medical and dental history. Diagnosis of periodontal diseases has the following concerns, which are among the main challenges in the field of periodontology:

- Detection of disease.
- Classification of disease categories (classification).
- Detection of disease activity.
- Prediction of disease onset (risk determination).
- Detection of early stage disease in clinically asymptomatic individuals (screening).
- Prediction of treatment outcomes (treatment planning).
- Detection of recurrence (monitoring).

Periodontal diagnosis should include an assessment of risk factors for periodontitis. A variety of systemic diseases and conditions interact with periodontitis or its treatment, and therefore, their screening should be part of a standard periodontal examination. The benefits of these records are two-fold; firstly possible risk factors for periodontal disease onset and progression can be identified and secondly undiagnosed systemic diseases and conditions can be diagnosed by referring the patient to the relevant physician. In this way, oral healthcare professionals would contribute to improve patients' oral and general health and have a more significant role in the wellbeing of the population (Glick et al. 2012).

The treatment plan of a periodontal patient usually relies on the clinical signs and symptoms of periodontal disease. Thus, the clinical diagnosis directly affects the decisions of the clinician to start therapy and select the relevant treatment modalities. The outcomes of clinical periodontal evaluations may be affected by various factors related to the clinician, the patient, or the nature of periodontal disease. Thus, the subjectivity of the clinical periodontal evaluations decreases the reproducibility and even the accuracy of the clinical diagnosis of a particular patient. Indeed, a very high heterogeneity in perceived risk for periodontal patients has been reported even among selected expert clinicians (Persson et al. 2003). Increasing the specificity and sensitivity of diagnostic tests may increase the long-term success of periodontal treatment thereby decreasing the treatment costs and improving the society's periodontal health state. The terms "specificity" and "sensitivity" were first described in Yerushalmy (1947) for dichotomous tests. High sensitivity is a desired property for a diagnostic test in order not to miss any positive cases, whereas high specificity is a desired property to avoid false positives. Preferentially, the predictive value of a diagnostic test should also be high and this value is closely related with the prevalence of the particular disease or condition in a particular population. Thus, the predictive value of a test may vary in a university clinic or even in a private office's patient portfolio compared to the general population. The prevalence would be higher among the individuals seeking treatment than the population in general. Similarly, it varies between the target populations of the primary and secondary prevention making the prevalence much higher in secondary prevention.

On the other hand, assessing a disease or health condition dichotomously as present or absent may be a too vague evaluation and may not provide appropriate data for a treatment plan. The dichotomizing cut-off levels are usually chosen or decided artificially in spite of the fact that most of the diagnostic parameters are continuous. Algorithms may help to evaluate the presence or absence of disease without imposing an arbitrary threshold (Pretty and Maupone 2004).

Conventional periodontal diagnosis is based on clinical and radiographical evaluations that mainly consist of measurement of probing depth and clinical attachment level, colour and contour changes, bleeding, gingival recession, suppuration, furcation lesions, and tooth mobility. Pocket formation and loss of attachment are pathognomonic for periodontal diseases. This reality spontaneously defines the clinical treatment goals as the reduction of probing depth and gain of attachment. Moreover, the utility, efficiency, and cost-effectiveness of the periodontal treatment are judged with these clinical parameters. The way a test or diagnostic algorithm performs in a specific patient and the consequences of a positive or negative test determines the capacity or potential of that diagnostic system. Evidence-based and well-defined information on the benefits and limitations of the available diagnostic methods may change clinical practice and eventually provide better therapeutic outcomes.

Presence or absence of bleeding on probing is a valuable clinical evaluation that continues to be the best negative predictor of periodontal disease activity, where its absence predicts lack of periodontal tissue destruction, yet it has low sensitivity value. Radiographs provide additional information on the location and extent of the disease and also about the neighbouring anatomical structures. However, all these parameters only give information about the history, the past disease activity, and previous destruction episodes (Buduneli and Kinane 2011). Therefore, they can be considered as retrospective diagnostic tools that neither tell about the current state nor predict the future in terms of disease progression, recurrence, or the response to treatment. On the other hand, knowing the disease activity or even better predicting sites that will lose attachment may help in early intervention and eventually saving more teeth may become possible. Early diagnosis and control of periodontal disease is the paramount goal for the clinician. As treatment of periodontitis is time-consuming and expensive, early detection and management are promising tools for considerable health-care benefits.

Presence or absence of microbial dental plaque is worth to be evaluated in each and every patient with a periodontal problem. This is the main parameter to assess the level of oral hygiene in a particular patient and this information is required also for the correct classification of the periodontal disease.

All these clinical periodontal parameters have their interim advantages and disadvantages. There are numerous index systems for each clinical periodontal parameter. Using index systems improves the objectivity, provides numerical data, and enables communication among dental professionals. The clinical data should be recorded on periodontal charts for clinical diagnosis and also for follow-up comparisons (Fig. 3.3).

Probing depth and clinical attachment level measurements in terms of millimetres are mandatory to discriminate gingivitis from periodontitis. The outcome of periodontal probing is affected by some factors such as the design of the probe tip, the pressure applied by the probe, the degree of inflammation in the soft tissue affecting its resistance, and the angulation of the probe. Periodontal probes can be manual, pressure sensitive, or computerised. The most commonly used ones are manual probes with variable design. Whether or not the clinician is experienced in terms of clinical sense is also important and may change the measurement to some extent. Another factor affecting the measurement outcome is the tolerance of the patient; some patients can be extremely sensitive showing signs of pain and this can prevent application of an appropriate probing force. It is clear that the measurement outcome by periodontal probe needs to be considered with precaution and both intra-examiner and inter-examiner calibrations are required particularly in clinical follow-up studies.

At this point, risk indicators need to be distinguished from the diagnostic factors. Presence of deep probing depths and/or increased clinical attachment level indicate a higher risk for progression as well as repopulation of pathogenic subgingival bacteria that will lead to recurrence of disease at certain sites. The American Academy of Periodontology states that risk assessment is increasingly important in periodontal treatment planning and should be part of every comprehensive dental and periodontal evaluation (AAP Guidelines 2006). Risk assessment is the deliberate

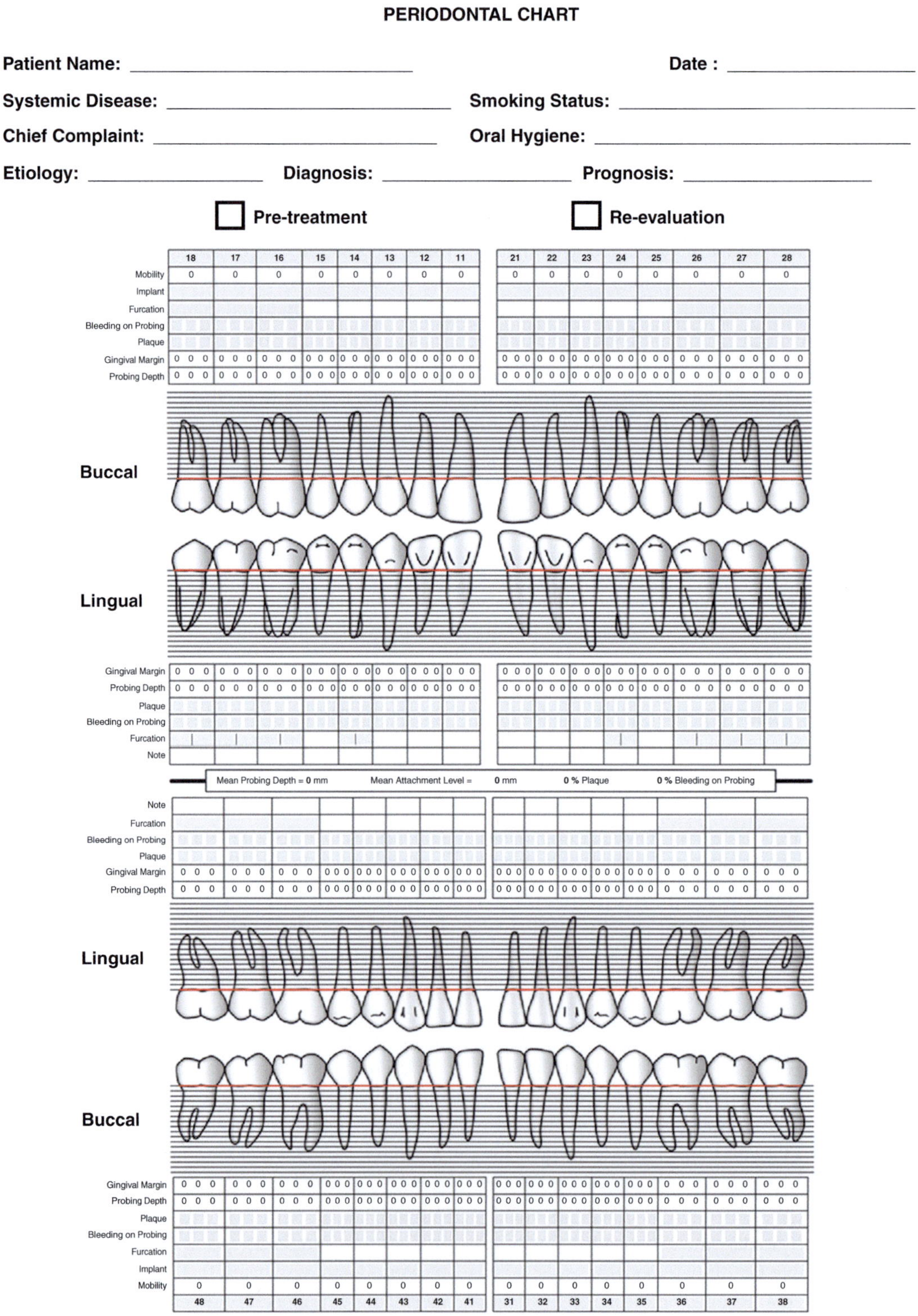

Fig. 3.3 An example of periodontal chart

and thoughtful evaluation of all circumstances that can affect the outcome of a therapeutic intervention (Armitage 2013). Risk factors may be either modifiable or nonmodifiable. The presence of risk factors increases the probability of a disease occurrence and their absence decreases the probability. They are usually part of, or expose the host to, the casual chain (Genco et al. 1996).

The clinical evaluations for periodontal diagnosis can be divided into three major categories as follows:

1. Evaluation of local etiological factors: using indices for assessment of oral hygiene; plaque indices.
2. Evaluation of inflammation: using indices of gingival bleeding.
3. Visual signs of periodontal tissue destruction: probing depth and clinical attachment level measurements.

3.5.1 Bleeding on Probing

The microulcerations in the inflamed gingiva cause bleeding during or immediately after probing with a periodontal probe (Fig. 3.4). Ulcerated, inflamed epithelium can be easily perforated by a periodontal probe and the fragile vessels are compressed or lacerated causing bleeding. The negative predictability of bleeding on probing is much higher than its positive predictability. However, smoking may suppress bleeding due to the vascular changes and whether or not the patient is a smoker should be considered while assessing the presence or absence of bleeding on probing.

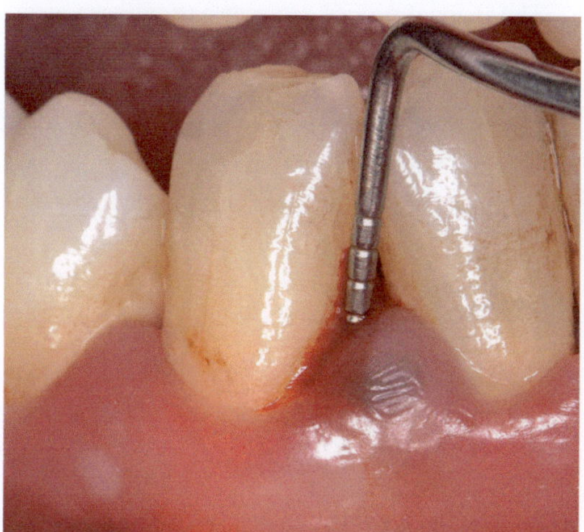

Fig. 3.4 Bleeding on probing; major sign of gingival inflammation

3.5.2 Suppuration

Pus or suppuration can be frequently present in severe periodontitis cases. The presence of abundant number of neutrophils in the gingival crevicular fluid transforms it into a purulent exudate (Armitage 1996). This sign is present only in a very low percentage (3–5%), and therefore, cannot be considered as a good indicator. The historical term of periodontitis "piorrea alveolaris" defines pus coming from periodontal pocket. Presence or absence of pus is usually examined by placing the ball of the index finger along the lateral aspect of the marginal gingiva and applying pressure in a rolling motion and apico-coronal direction.

Calibrated periodontal probe has been a routine part of periodontal treatment for almost a century now. Periodontal probes are used to measure probing depth, clinical attachment level, and relative attachment level. Gingival margin is located approximately 1–3 mm coronal to the cementoenamel junction in normal (intact) and healthy periodontium. Presence of oedema, gingival enlargement, or gingival recession may cause shifts in the position of free gingival margin (Fig. 3.5).

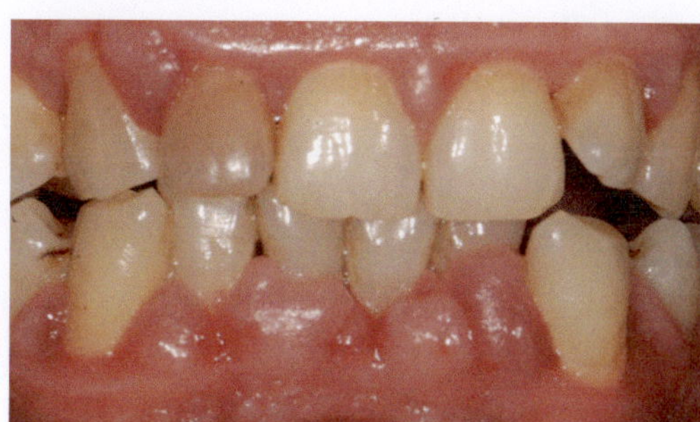

Fig. 3.5 Gingival hyperplasia and oedema due to longstanding inflammation

3.5.3 Clinical Attachment Level

This term indicates the distance between the cementoenamel junction and the base of the pocket that is the most coronal part of the junctional epithelium. This measurement indicates the portion of the lost connective tissue attachment and indirectly reveals the existing periodontal attachment.

3.5.4 Relative Attachment Level

In cases where the cementoenamel junction cannot be identified, the reference point can be a restoration border or another fixed point. The distance from this reference point to the base of the pocket is measured by a periodontal probe and it is called as the relative attachment level.

3.5.5 Probing Depth

The pocket depth means either biological (histological) pocket depth or clinical (probing) pocket depth. They are not necessarily the same. Probing depth shows the distance that is measured by a calibrated periodontal probe from the free gingival margin to the base of the pocket that is the most coronal part of the junctional epithelium. The probe should be inserted parallel to the long axis of the tooth and "walked" circumferentially around each surface of each tooth not to miss narrow but deep pockets.

Factors affecting the outcome of periodontal probing (Box 3.1).

Box 3.1 Factors Affecting Probing Outcome

- Design of the probe tip
- Angulation of the probe
- Probing force applied
- Tissue inflammation

- The diameter of the probe tip: The thinner the probe tip is, the further distance it can reach and the measured value becomes larger.
- The pressure applied during probing: The greater the probing force, the deeper the penetration of the probe into the tissue. The optimal probing force is 0.5–0.75 N. The pressure sensitive probes enable the clinician to probe with a predetermined force but still there is a risk of over- or under-estimation of the true pocket depth or attachment level.
- The degree of inflammation in the soft tissue: Compared to the healthy tissue, the inflamed tissue contains more inflammatory cells and less collagen that makes it less resistant towards mechanical forces and this can lead larger measurements. Smoking suppresses gingival inflammation and this reduced inflammation in smokers prevents easy penetration of the periodontal probe tip enabling a more accurate measurement of probing depth in smokers compared to non-smokers (Biddle et al. 2001).
- The angulation of the probe: Ideally the probe should be placed parallel to the long axis of the tooth and wrong angulations may cause erroneous measurements. Malposition of the probe due to anatomic features such as the contour of the tooth surface may not permit appropriate angulation of the probe and result in erroneous measurements.

The manual probes can measure with an accuracy of ±1 mm. There are manual periodontal probes with different design and markings (Fig. 3.6). The accuracy of pressure sensitive probes or computerised probes is 0.1 mm. However, computerised probes lack the tactile sense and the patient comfort is worse compared to the manual probes.

Visual signs of periodontal tissue destruction are:

- Morphological changes in gingival tissue (changes in colour, contours, size, consistency, position).
- Gingival recession.
- Increased mobility.
- Furcation lesions.
- Tooth migration.

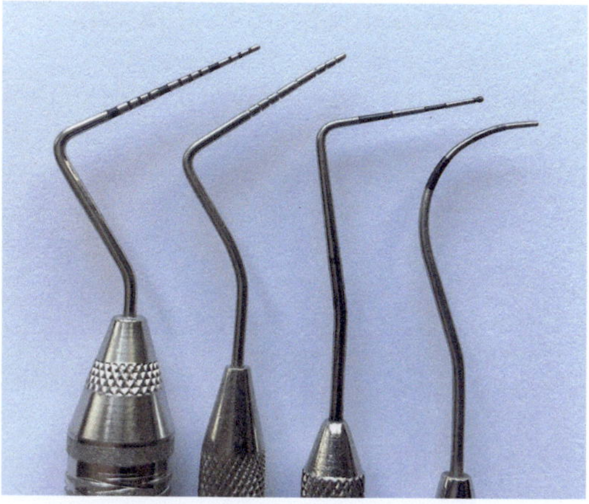

Fig. 3.6 Manual probes with various designs (from left to the right: UNC15 probe, Williams probe, WHO probe, Nabers probe)

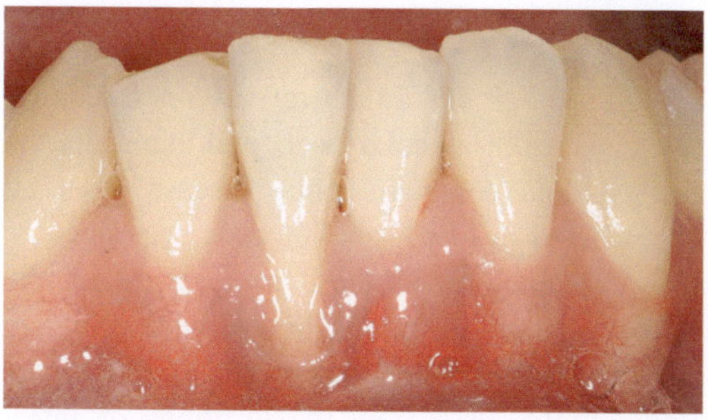

Fig. 3.7 Localised gingival recession affecting lower right central incisor

Loss of papillae and formation of interdental craters are usually signs of necrotising periodontal diseases. Thickening of gingival margins and blunt appearance are due to long-standing gingival inflammation.

3.5.6 Gingival Recession

This parameter indicates the distance between the gingival margin and the cementoenamel junction (Fig. 3.7). The apically displacement of the free gingival margin is clearly a sign of attachment loss. However, it is not necessarily due to periodontitis. Common causes of gingival recession are anatomical factors such as crowding of teeth, improper ratio of root/alveolar crest width, thin phenotype (formerly called as thin biotype), and traumatic tooth brushing.

3.5.7 Furcation Lesions

When periodontal disease around multi-rooted teeth progresses, the destructive process may involve the supporting structures of the furcation area. Furcation lesions are difficult to access sites not only for the patient but also for the clinician, and therefore, they are problematic. The early diagnosis of furcation involvement is of utmost importance for successful treatment outcomes. The precise identification of the presence and extent of furcation lesions need meticulous vertical and horizontal probing. Specific periodontal probes such as Nabers probe are required for horizontal probing of the furcation area.

3.5.8 Pathologic Tooth Migration

Alterations in tooth position should be carefully noted and presence of abnormal forces, tongue-thrusting habit, or other possible contributing habits should be investigated. Pathologic migration of anterior teeth in young people is usually a sign of severe periodontitis. When the functional forces exceed the tolerance limit of periodontal tissues, the tooth can become hypermobile or migrate in the alveolus. A tooth may lose its original position if there is severe loss of bone and attachment. Although it is a late sign of advanced periodontitis, tooth migration is among the major symptoms that make the patient seek treatment.

3.5.9 Increased Tooth Mobility

Orthodontic treatment or dentures may cause excessive functional forces, occlusal trauma and endodontic or periodontal problems may cause alveolar bone resorption and severe resorption may cause increased tooth mobility. The underlying factor of increased mobility must be carefully evaluated, as it does not have to be periodontitis. First the clinical attachment level should be measured. If there is no or very little attachment loss, then causes other than periodontitis should be looked for. Increased mobility does not necessarily affect the prognosis in an adverse way. The critical factor is the level of oral hygiene. Following a successful periodontal treatment, hypermobility may remain persistent, but it should be investigated meticulously whether there is a progressive increase in the mobility. The severity of tooth mobility can be measured by a specific instrument (Periotest®). This instrument applies percussion to the tooth four times per second and electronically records the reaction of the tooth to these forces.

3.5.10 Bone Sounding

Bone sounding can be performed by inserting the periodontal probe tip into the pocket following local anaesthesia. The probe tip is forced through the supraalveolar connective tissue to make contact with the bone and the distance from the cementoenamel junction to the bone level is measured in mm.

3.5.11 Oral Hygiene Status

The basic clinical periodontal examination should always include assessment of the patient's oral hygiene status. Presence or absence of microbial dental plaque/oral biofilm should be investigated on each tooth surface. Disclosing solutions may be used to facilitate their detection particularly to show the patient or just visual examination by the help of a periodontal probe may be preferred. Retentive factors such as overhanging restorations, supra and subgingival calculus should also be identified for a proper clinical periodontal examination and accurate clinical diagnosis. Supragingival calculus can be directly seen and subgingival calculus should be carefully searched by an explorer.

3.6 Radiographical Evaluation

Intraoral (periapical, bite-wing) or extraoral (panoramic) radiographs provide additional information on the height and configuration of the alveolar bone (Box 3.2).

Box 3.2 Radiographs Frequently Used for Periodontal Purposes

Dental radiographs

- Intraoral radiographs
  - Periapical radiograph
  - Bitewing radiograph
- Extraoral radiographs
  - Panoramic radiography

The radiographs do not reveal minor destructive changes in alveolar bone, and therefore, the earliest signs of periodontal disease must be investigated by clinical parameters. Developmental anomalies, pathologies of the teeth, jaws, and the temporomandibular joint can be detected in the panoramic radiographs. Radiographs also show the locations of interproximal calculus, but this is not a valid objective for obtaining radiographs. The additional information that can be obtained by radiographs can be outlined as follows:

- The amount of bone loss: The radiographs show the remaining amount bone and then the lost bone amount can be determined.
- The distribution of bone loss: Particularly panoramic radiographs provide information on the location of bone destruction.
- The type of bone loss: Alveolar bone loss can be horizontal, vertical, or circumferential or sometimes a combination of these can be present.
- The distance of the periodontal lesion to the adjacent anatomical structures: This information can only be obtained by radiographs and examples of such anatomical structures are foramen mentale or mandibular canal.

- The degree of furcation lesions: The definitive diagnosis of furcation lesions is made by clinical detection methods, but radiolucency in the furcation area may alert the clinician for special focus. As a general rule, bone loss is always greater than it appears in the radiograph.
- Presence of periapical pathologies: Periapical lesions, cysts, or granulomas can be detected in radiographs and these lesions can be in contact with periodontal lesions.
- The aetiology of bone resorption: The location of destructive local factors can be investigated by observing the distribution of bone loss.

3.7 Limitations of the Conventional Diagnostic Methods

The clinical periodontal examination is basic and mandatory for each and every patient. However, the clinical periodontal parameters have their limitations and disadvantages together with their advantages (Box 3.3). First of all, these clinical parameters provide information about the past and without standardised and long-term measurements, they hardly give information about the present or future of the disease. The sensitivity and specificity of clinical periodontal parameters are rather low. There is no way to determine either the risk or the presence of current disease activity at a single visit. Another important limitation is that there should be significant amount of damage so that the clinical evaluation method can detect it and provide information about the severity of the periodontal destruction. Furthermore, there is always some extent of subjectivity in the measurement of each clinical parameter and without inter- and intra-examiner calibration; there is a risk of great variability in the recordings making the reproducibility and accuracy of these measurements questionable and leading inconsistent diagnoses.

Box 3.3 The Limitations of Clinical Periodontal Indices

Clinical periodontal indices

- Low sensitivity and specificity
- Subjective
- Questionable reproducibility
- Shows history
- No clue on progression, treatment efficacy

3.8 Conclusion

As a conclusion, it is quite clear that more precise diagnostic tools and methods are needed for more accurate and early diagnosis and also for monitoring patients with periodontal diseases. Clinical index systems are mandatory to use (Box 3.4).

Box 3.4 The Reasons Why We Need the Index Systems

Why do we need index systems?

- For quantitative evaluation
- To decrease subjectivity
- For reproducible assessment
- For communication among dental professionals

Given the complex nature of periodontitis, it is unlikely that one single clinical or laboratory examination can address all issues concerning diagnosis, classification, and prognosis (Van der Velden 2005; Xiang et al. 2010). Certainly, there are characteristics sought in an ideal index system (Fig. 3.8).

One of the characteristics of periodontal diseases is the lack of pain, apart from very limited acute problems such as acute necrotising ulcerative gingivitis and acute periodontal abscess, pain is not the sign or symptom forcing the patient to seek treatment. The insidious nature of chronic periodontal diseases retards the diagnosis and intervention unless the patient is under a regular control program. Development of such techniques or tests with high sensitivity and specificity may help to make individually tailored treatment

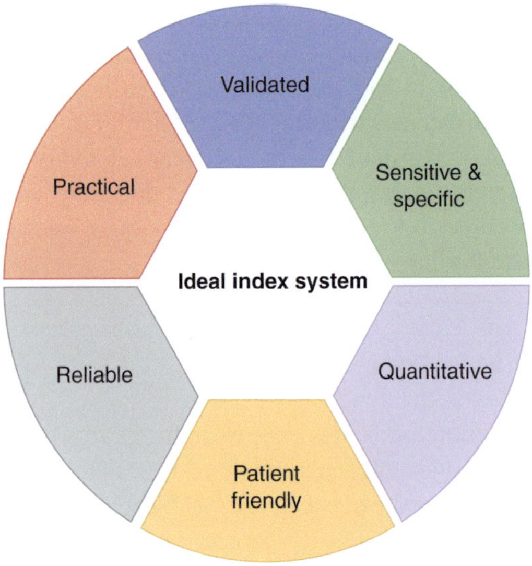

Fig. 3.8 Characteristics of an ideal index system for periodontal diagnosis

plan not only for a particular patient but also for a particular tooth or site. Saving more teeth for a lifetime can then become a reality for much more people in the world. An ideal periodontal diagnostic method should be able firstly to screen susceptible subjects in the general population, secondly to differentiate active sites from inactive sites and thirdly to predict future tissue destruction on patient- and site-based and finally to monitor the response to periodontal therapy (Buduneli and Kinane 2011).

References

American Academy of Periodontology. Discussion section I. Periodontal diagnosis and diagnostic aids. Proceedings of the World Workshop in Clinical Periodontics. Consensus Report, Princeton: American Academy of Periodontology; 1989.

American Academy of Periodontology. Guidelines for the management of patients with periodontal diseases. J Periodontol. 2006;77:1607–11.

Armitage RC. Periodontal diseases: Diagnosis. Ann Periodontol. 1996;1:37–215.

Armitage RC. Development of a classification system for periodontal diseases and conditions. Ann Periodontol. 1999;4:1–6.

Armitage RC. Classifying periodontal diseases—a long-standing dilemma. Periodontology. 2002;30:9–23.

Armitage GC. Learned and unlearned concepts in periodontal diagnostics: a 50-year perspective. Periodontology. 2013;62:20–36.

Biddle AJ, Palmer RM, Wilson RF, Watts TL. Comparison of the validity of periodontal probing measurements in smokers and non-smokers. J Clin Periodontol. 2001;28:806–12.

Buduneli N, Kinane DF. Host-derived diagnostic markers related to soft tissue destruction and bone degradation in periodontitis. J Clin Periodontol. 2011;38(Suppl.11):85–105.

Genco RJ, Jeffcoat M, JJr C, et al. Consensus report: periodontal diseases: epidemiology and diagnosis. Ann Periodontol. 1996;1:216–22.

Glick M, Monteiro da Silva O, Seeberger GK, et al. FDI vision 2020: shaping the future of oral health. Int Dent J. 2012;62:278–91.

Gold SI. Periodontics—the past. Part (I) early sources. J Clin Periodontol. 1985;12:79–97.

Gottlieb B. Zur aetiologie und therapie der alveolarporrhoe. Z Stomatol. 1920;18:59–82.

Gottlieb B. Die diffuse atrophie des alveolar knochens. Z Stomatol. 1923;31:195–201.

Gottlieb B. The formation of the pocket: diffuse atrophy of alveolar bone. J Am Dent Assoc. 1928;15:462–76.

Graetz C, Mann L, Krois J, Salzer S, Kahl M, Springer C, Schwendicke F. Comparison of periodontitis patients' classification in the 2018 versus 1999 classification. J Clin Periodontol. 2019;46:908–17.

McCall JO, Box HK. The pathology and diagnosis of the basic lesions of chronic periodontitis. J Am Dent Assoc. 1925;12:1300–9.

Page RC, Schroeder HE. Current status of the host response in chronic marginal periodontitis. J Periodontol. 1981;52:477–91.

Papapanou PN, Sanz M, Buduneli N, et al. Periodontitis: consensus report of workgroup 2 of the 2017 world workshop on the classification of periodontal and peri-implant diseases and conditions. J Clin Periodontol. 2018;45(Suppl 20):S162–70.

Persson GR, Mancl LA, Martin J, Page RC. Assessing periodontal disease risk: a comparison of clinicians' assessment versus a computerised tool. J Am Dent Assoc. 2003;134:575–82.

Pretty IA, Maupone GA. Closer look at diagnosis in clinical dental practice: part 2. Using predictive values and receiver operating characteristics in assessing diagnostic accuracy. J Can Dent Assoc. 2004;70:313–6.

Tonetti MS, Greenwell H, Kornman KS. Staging and grading of periodontitis: framework and proposal of a new classification and case definition. J Clin Periodontol. 2018;45(Suppl 20):S149–61.

Van der Velden. Purpose and problems of periodontal disease classification. Periodontology. 2005;39:13–21.

van der Velden U. What exactly distinguishes aggressive from chronic periodontitis: Is it mainly a difference in the degree of bacterial invasiveness? Periodontol 2000. 2017;75:24–44.

Xiang X, Sowa MG, Iacopino AM, et al. An update on novel non-invasive approaches for periodontal diagnosis. J Periodontol. 2010;81:186–98.

Yerushalmy J. Statistical problems in assessing methods of medical diagnosis, with special reference to X-ray techniques. Public Health Rep. 1947;62:1432–49.

4 Novel Diagnostic Approaches in Periodontics

During the last 50 years significant technical developments took place in the field of periodontal diagnosis. Untreated periodontal diseases may cause tooth loss and create functional, social, aesthetical, and self-esteem problems lowering the quality of life. The proper management of periodontal diseases requires a correct and timely diagnosis as a first step. Clinical periodontal evaluations continue to be the basic and mandatory tools to have a diagnosis, evaluate prognosis, and make a treatment plan. Recording whole-mouth clinical periodontal parameters on periodontal charts is time-consuming and requires an assisting person. Considering the subjectivity and possible errors in this conventional method, researchers have developed novel technologies to make the periodontal investigation easier, faster, and more precise. To overcome the inherent problems of manual periodontal probes pressure-sensitive probes and automated digital probes have been developed. Moreover, in order to make the recording easier, voice-activated recording systems are now available for the dental practitioners.

Radiographic evaluation provides valuable additional information when coupled with clinical periodontal parameters. Two-dimensional radiographs can be easily reached, are cost-effective and have high resolution. 2D systems use image receptors like radiographic films or intensifying screens. These include periapical views, panoramic, occlusal, and cephalometric radiography. A digital 2D image is described by an image matrix that has individual picture elements called pixels. Each pixel has discrete digital value that describes image intensity at a particular point (Hausmann 2000).

Periapical views depict severe alveolar bone loss, but distort the location of bone height along the tooth root and do not reveal the osseous crest precisely, cannot detect moderate periodontal bone loss. On the contrary, bitewings can assess bone height in patients with moderate to severe bone loss (Jeffcoat et al. 1995). Panoramic view is commonly used in today's dental practice and provides an overall view of the periodontium, thereby minimises the radiation exposure, but the image distortion is a shortcoming (Eley and Cox 1998).

2D systems have limitations like being dependent on the observer's eyes and underestimating bone loss due to projection errors (Benn 1990; Bragger 2005). Particularly, defects on the straight buccal or palatal sides and furcation defects may be difficult to detect using the 2-dimensional radiographs.

There are also advanced 2D imaging techniques such as xeroradiography that is an excellent aid evaluating initial osseous changes, assessment of osseous repair after periodontal therapy, and clearly visualises the crestal dimensions (Lopez 1976). Another example is stereoscopy, which can be used for the assessment of infrabony pockets, but needs long exposure time

N. Buduneli, *Biomarkers in Periodontal Health and Disease*,
https://doi.org/10.1007/978-3-030-37317-7_4

(White and Pharaoh White and Pharaoh 2004a, b). There is scenography (soredex scanora) that performs rotational and linear imaging and the rotational scenography is capable of assessing periodontal disease (White and Pharaoh White and Pharaoh 2004a, b).

4.1 Controlled-Force, Standardised Probes

The periodontal probe is the most commonly used diagnostic tool for diagnosis as well as screening and monitoring of periodontal diseases. However, the problems posed by conventional periodontal probing may lead erroneous diagnosis and/or categorisation of the disease. For many years now, investigators have sought a more precise method for measuring probing depth and attachment level with much smaller thresholds and much higher accuracy. The automated probes are among these considerably novel techniques. They apply controlled force, they provide direct computer input, and reference landmark recognition for relative or clinical attachment measurements. The automated Florida probe greatly reduces measurement error and can detect a loss of attachment level of less than 1 mm change with a certainty of 99% (Gibbs et al. 1988). The Florida Probe uses a reproducible occlusal landmark or a customised stent margin as a reference landmark. The Foster-Miller probe registers the cementoenamel junction as its attachment level landmark. This latter probe was suggested to be able to determine clinical attachment levels with a repeatability of 0.2 mm in an in vitro study. The computerised probes have the advantage of directly transferring the data to the computer for statistical software analysis. Conventional manual periodontal probes are in routine use worldwide, but they require at least 2 mm change in attachment level so that the clinician can identify sites loosing attachment. Computerised probes can detect much smaller changes and their usage should shorten the interval between two control visits, leading to earlier diagnosis and intervention. However, in spite of these advantages, computerised probes could not become a routine part of the periodontal examination so far. The major reasons behind may be their high cost and the need of the clinician for technical training to be competent in using these probes.

4.2 Voice-Activated Charting System

This system makes recording of full-mouth clinical periodontal parameters easier and faster. As the charting becomes more practical, more patients would feel comfortable during the screening and more dental professionals would use the charting routinely and screening would be well accepted.

4.3 Advanced Techniques with 3-Dimensional Imaging

These techniques promise more accurate and detailed topographic information on bone defects as well as anatomical structures.

Similar to the conventional probes, conventional radiographs can detect progressing bone loss when two or more standardised radiographs are obtained and compared. However, the change either in the height or configuration of alveolar bone must be big enough to be detected. Conventional radiographs only demonstrate alveolar bone loss when 30–50% of bone mineral in a specific area is destroyed (Jeffcoat 1992). For conventional radiographs, this may take several months to occur. Moreover, the 2-dimensional radiographs have disadvantages, such as overlapping of anatomical structures, difficulty of standardisation, and underestimation of periodontal bone defect dimensions (Haas et al. 2018). Conventional radiography offers reliable, low dose procedures and digital imaging per se is not superior to film-based radiographs in the detailed depiction of periodontal structures.

Technical improvements are required to be able to detect small changes and take precautions before too much attachment is lost and too much bone is resorbed. The main difficulty of radiographic interpretation is demarcating the pathology from the normal anatomic background. The irrelevant structures are called as "noise". Noise elimination is possible by subtraction radiography.

4.4 Computer-Assisted Digital Radiography

Subtraction radiography technique can automatically compare two standardised radiographs taken with a time interval and detect small amounts of positive or negative changes. A subtraction image, subtracts the background features, minimises background complexity, and amplifies even minor density differences by superimposing serial images obtained at consecutive sessions. It uses colour coding as shades of red (indicating loss of bone) and green (indicating gain of bone). Digital subtraction radiography can detect early changes in alveolar bone such as 1–5% per unit volume of bone is lost. Major limitations of this technique are the need for accurate alignment during sequential radiographic exposures, essential prerequisites like reproducible exposure geometry, identical contrast, and density of the serial radiographs (Fidler et al. 2000). This technique is highly sensitive to any physical noise occurring between radiographs and minor changes lead to large errors in the results (Kornman 1987). Differences in image contrast and intensity between baseline and follow-ups can hamper the detection and make the quantitative findings unreliable (White and Phoraoh White and Pharaoh 2004a, b). Hence, this technique could not become part of the routine periodontics, but rather is being preferred for research purposes.

4.5 Computer-Assisted Densitometric Image Analysis (CADIA)

This is a modification of subtraction radiography and it gives precise information on the longitudinal changes in bone density that is very important in treatment procedures aiming bone regeneration. This technique is based on the comparison of two serial images obtained with standardised projection geometry and equalised for the density differences in the images. It can measure the area of change and the depth of lesion in a buccolingual plane (Bragger et al. 1988).

Computerised tomography (CT) as an imaging technique has been in the field of dentistry for many years now. CT is a specialised radiographic technique that portrays cross-sectional image of an object without superimposition of structures in the plane parallel to the X-ray beam. It is supposed to be 100 times more sensitive than conventional X-ray systems. There are different variants with individual focuses; cone-beam computed tomography (CBCT), quantitative computed tomography (QCT), tuned aperture computed tomography (TACT), and micro focus computed tomography (micro focus CT).

4.6 Cone-Beam Computerised Tomography

CBCT imaging is a powerful tool allowing for diagnosis of 3-dimensional structures and is well documented for accurate quantification and locating anatomic structures. It has no anatomical overlapping problem, it is relatively accessible and its radiation dose is lower than that of medical CT. Its radiation dose is equivalent to a full-mouth periapical series and approximately 3–7 times the dose of a panoramic radiograph, depending on the setting (Ludlow et al. 2006). CBCT was reported to be superior to the intraoral radiographs in terms of detecting furcation lesions (94.8% and 75.6%, respectively) and intrabony defects (99.7% and 82.7%, respectively) (Braun et al. 2014). Detection rates of dehiscence and fenestration defects were reported to be higher with CBCT (Bagis et al. 2015). The sensitivity of CBCT for the detection of bone defects varies between 80% and 100%, whereas this ratio is 63% and 67% with intraoral radiographs (Misch et al. 2006; Vandenberghe et al. 2007). Padmanabhan et al. (2017) reported that there was no statistical significance between CBCT and direct intra-surgical measurements regarding furcation height, width, and depth. CBCT is also beneficial in assessing root concavities of first premolars and associated pattern of bone loss (Zhao et al. 2014). CBCT can be also used for evaluation of phenotype by measuring hard and soft tissue thickness of the alveolar process. One of the best application ways for CBCT is the postoperative evaluation of the surgical site. Traditionally, this investigation is done by re-entry, which is invasive, time-consuming, and costly. American Academy of Periodontology recommended CBCT evaluation following regenerative surgical treatment of furcation lesions (Reddy et al. 2015). However, recently AAP released a best of evidence consensus (BEC) series of papers related to the use and application of CBCT in the field of periodontics. It was concluded that the evidence to support routine use of CBCT in the diagnosis, treatment planning, and management of periodontal disease was limited (Kim and Bassir 2017; McAllister and Eshraghi 2017). It is the responsibility of the clinician to determine whether or not to use CBCT and application of "As Low As Reasonably Achievable" (ALARA) principle. Even though CBCT exposures are considered as low exposure, if the information from an additional CBCT is not vital, it would not follow the ALARA principle. In a recent systematic review, Choi et al. (2018) concluded that CBCT is the best imaging technique to assess infrabony defects, furcation lesions, the height of the alveolar bone crest, and the periodontal ligament space. Mandelaris et al. (2017) stated that evidence from mainly observational studies (cohort and case series) supports the use of CBCT in dental implant patients for tasks such as evaluation of root morphology and associated pathology for extractions and reconstruction, location of relevant anatomic structures and their relation to implant placement, etc. CBCT also has a potential in patients, who require tooth movement. The best appealing indications for CBCT in regard with periodontitis were outlined as follows in the same paper (Mandelaris et al. 2017):

- When an advanced furcation lesion has been detected and dental implants are being considered as an alternative treatment option.
- When advanced bone loss has encroached on anatomic structures, such as sinus cavities or the inferior alveolar nerve.
- When there is a questionable root fracture, root resorption, or periodontal-endodontic lesion present that could not be identified by 2D imaging and/or clinical evaluation.
- In the treatment of cases that do not respond favourably to localised periodontal therapy.
- To enhance the diagnosis and management of peri-implantitis when determined necessary.

There are limitations of CBCT such as the larger the field of view the greater the amount of noise in the image. On the other hand, the smaller the size of the voxel, the best spatial resolution of the image, which allows visualisation of the bone tissue in areas with smaller thicknesses or lower bone density, e.g., on the base of defects containing demineralised bone tissue (Haas et al. 2018). Moreover, the presence of metallic materials in the oral cavity interferes with the diagnostic process performed on CBCT. The artefacts created by these materials are also defined as "missing value artefacts", and they reduce image quality (Schulze et al. 2011). The high cost and higher radiation of CBCT compared to the conventional 2-dimensional radiography limit its usage for cases when it would significantly benefit the patient if the diagnosis and decision-making are challenging by conventional diagnostics (Haas et al. 2018; Schmidt et al. 2019).

TACT is helpful in diagnosing crown or root fractures as well as detecting periodontal bone loss or gain, and alveolar contours (Webber et al. 1997). Cone-beam volumetric tomography (CBVT) is another variant of CT that obtains 3D images. It produces images that have high resolution and accuracy for measuring regenerative therapy outcomes following regenerative periodontal surgeries and indicates direct bone fill and defect resolution (Grimard et al. 2009). When CBVT is used for the evaluation of bone after treatment, there is no need for re-entry. QCT offers precise 3D anatomic localisation of bone density measurements in Hounsfield units (Shahlaie et al. 2003). Cortical and cancellous bone segments can be differentiated by QCT. Microfocus CT is a rather recent technique, which has a special resolution of <10 μm to evaluate trabecular bone structure (Rüegsegger et al. 1996; Ohta et al. 1999). This technique enables visualisation of fine trabecular pattern of newly formed bone (Kiba et al. 2003) and has the advantages such as easy and fast reconstruction of 3D images and minimal artefacts. Microfocus CT analysis enables highly quantitative and qualitative measurement of bone augmentation. Hence, it is a dynamic non-invasive method for measuring bone regeneration (Chakrapani et al. 2013).

4.7 Conclusion

Technological advances in the field of imaging techniques provide more precise and accurate methods for diagnosis of periodontal diseases. Early detection of periodontitis and intrabony defects may enable early intervention improving success of periodontal treatment. However, much progress is required in these imaging techniques to make them part of routine periodontal practice.

References

Bagis N, Kolsuz ME, Kursun S, Orhan K. Comparison of intraoral radiography and cone-beam computed tomography for the detection of periodontal defects: an in vitro study. BMC Oral Health. 2015;15:64.

Benn DK. A review of the reliability of radiographic measurements in estimating alveolar bone changes. J Clin Periodontol. 1990;17:14–21.

Bragger U. Radiographic parameters: biological significance and clinical use. Periodontol 2000. 2005;39:73–90.

Bragger U, Pasquali L, Rylander H, Carnes D, Kornman KS. Computer-assisted densitometric image analysis in periodontal radiography. A methodological study. J Clin Periodontol. 1988;15:27–30.

Braun X, Ritter L, Jervoe-Storm P-M, Frentzen M. Diagnostic accuracy of CBCT for periodontal lesions. Clin Oral Invest. 2014;18:1229–36.

Chakrapani S, Sirisha K, Srilalitha A, Srinivas M. Choice of diagnostic and therapeutic imaging in periodontics and implantology. J Indian Soc Periodontol. 2013;17:711–8.

Choi IGG, Cortes ARG, Arita ES, Georgetti MAP. Comparison of conventional imaging techniques and CBCT for periodontal evaluation: a systematic review. Imaging Sci Dent. 2018;48:79–86.

Eley BM, Cox SW. Advances in periodontal diagnosis. 1. Traditional clinical methods of diagnosis. Br Dent J. 1998;184:12–6.

Fidler A, Likar B, Pernus F, Skaleric U. Influence of developer exhaustion on accuracy of quantitative digital subtraction radiography: An in vitro study. Oral Surg Oral Med Oral Pathol Oral Radion Endod. 2000;90:233–9.

Gibbs CH, Hisrchfeld JW, Lee JG, et al. Description and clinical evaluation of a new computerised periodontal probe-the Florida probe. J Clin Periodontol. 1988;15:137–44.

Grimard BA, Hoidal MJ, Mills MP, Mellonig JT, Nummikoski PV, Mealey BL. Comparison of clinical, periapical radiograph, and cone-beam volume tomography measurement techniques for assessing bone level changes following regenerative periodontal therapy. J Periodontol. 2009;80:48–55.

Haas LF, Zimmermann GS, Canto GDL, Flores-Mir C, Correa M. Precision of cone beam CT to assess periodontal bone defects: a systematic review and meta-analysis. Dentomaxillofac Radiol. 2018;47:20170084.

Hausmann E. Radiographic and digital imaging in periodontal practice. J Periodontol. 2000;71:497–503.

Jeffcoat MK. Radiographic methods for the detection of progressive alveolar bone loss. J Periodontol. 1992;63(Suppl 4):367–72.

Jeffcoat MK, Wang IC, Reddy MS. Radiographic diagnosis in periodontics. Periodontol 2000. 1995;7:54–68.

Kiba H, Hayakawa T, Oba S, Kuwabara M, Habata I, Yamamoto H. Potential application of high-resolution microfocus X-ray techniques for observation of bone structure and bone-implant interface. Int J Oral Maxillofac Implants. 2003;18:279–85.

Kim DM, Bassir SH. When is cone-beam computed tomography imaging appropriate for diagnostic inquiry in the management of inflammatory periodontitis? An American Academy of Periodontology Best Evidence Review. J Periodontol. 2017;88:978–98.

Kornman KS. Nature of periodontal diseases: assessment and diagnosis. J Periodontal Res. 1987;22:192–204.

Lopez J Jr. Xeroradiography in dentistry. J Am Dent Assoc. 1976;92:106–10.

Ludlow JB, Davies-Ludlow LE, Brooks SL, Howerton WB. Dosimetry of 3 CBCT devices for oral and maxillofacial radiology: CB Mercuray, NewTom 3G and i-CAT. Dentomaxillofac Radiol. 2006;35:219–26.

Mandelaris GA, Scheyer ET, Evans M, et al. American academy of periodontology best evidence statement on selected oral applications cone-beam computed tomography. J Periodontol. 2017;88:939–45.

McAllister BS, Eshraghi VT. Commentary: cone-beam computed tomography: an essential technology for management of complex periodontal and implant cases. J Periodontol. 2017;88:937–8.

Misch KA, Yi ES, Sarment DP. Accuracy of cone beam computed tomography for periodontal defect measurements. J Periodontol. 2006;77:1261–6.

Ohta T, Harada Y, Yamada N, Takagi H, Azuma Y, Komoriya K. Three dimensional analysis of bone structure by microfocus X-ray computed tomography. J Soc Bone Morphometry. 1999;9:97–101.

Padmanabhan S, Dommy A, Guru SR, Joseph A. Comparative evaluation of cone-beam computed tomography versus direct surgical measurements in the diagnosis of mandibular molar furcation involvement. Contemp Clin Dent. 2017;8:439–45.

Reddy MS, Aichelmann-Reidy ME, Avila-Ortiz G, et al. Periodontal regeneration-furcation defects: a consensus report from the AAP regeneration workshop. J Periodontol. 2015;86:S131–3.

Rüegsegger P, Koller B, Müller R. A microtomographic system for the non-destructive evaluation of bone architecture. Calcif Tissue Int. 1996;58:24–9.

Schmidt JC, Gutekunst C-J, Dagassan-Berndt D, Schmidlin PR, Walter C. Comparison of two-dimensional and three-dimensional radiographs using clinically relevant parameters. Dent J. 2019;7:50.

Schulze R, Heil U, Gross D, et al. Artefacts in CBCT: a review. Dentomaxillofac Radiol. 2011;40:265–73.

Shahlaie M, Gantes B, Schulz E, Riggs M, Crigger M. Bone density assessments of dental implant sites: 1 Quantitative computed tomography. Int J Oral Maxillofac Implants. 2003;18:224–31.

Vandenberghe B, Jacobs R, Yang J. Diagnostic validity (or acuity) of 2D CCD versus 3D CBCT-images for assessing periodontal breakdown. Oral Surg Oral Med Oral Pathol Oral Radiol Endod. 2007;104:395–401.

Webber RL, Horton RA, Tyndall DA, Ludlow JB. Tuned-aperture computed tomography (TACT). Theory and application for three-dimensional dento-alveolar imaging. Dentomaxillofac Radiol. 1997;26:53–62.

White SC, Pharaoh MJ. Oral radiology principles and interpretation. 5th ed. St.Louis, MO: Mosby Publication; 2004a. p. 225–45.

White SC, Pharaoh MJ. Oral radiology principles and interpretation. 5th ed. St.Louis, MO: Mosby Publication; 2004b. p. 248–50.

Zhao H, Wang H, Pan Y, Pan C, Jin X. The relationship between root concavities in first premolars and chronic periodontitis. J Periodontal Res. 2014;49:213–9.

Biomarkers for Periodontal Diseases

5

5.1 Main Text

5.1.1 How to Find a Needle in the Haystack?

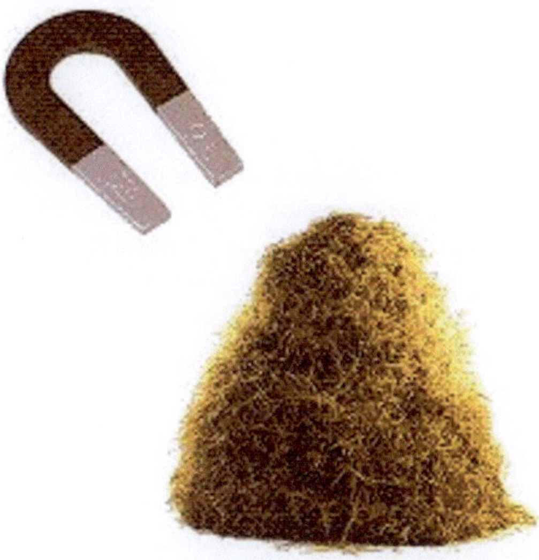

Periodontitis is the sixth most common chronic inflammatory disease in the world (Kassebaum et al. 2014). Technological progress together with advances in diagnostic research is promising for the development of methods to identify individual periodontal risk and quantify the risk by objective biomarkers (Taba et al. 2005). Biomarker research aims to find reliable markers for the present and future states of periodontal disease (Özmeriç 2014). A variety of diagnostic tests basing on physical, chemical, microbiological, and immunological methodologies have been documented in the last two decades (Curtis et al. 1989; Kinane 2009). There is a high level of demand but also the expectations are high from candidate biomarkers to be used for periodontal diseases (Fig. 5.1).

One of the main challenges in the field of periodontology is to discover an ideal periodontal diagnostic/prognostic biomarker, which would be able to achieve the following goals:

1. to identify current disease activity
2. to differentiate active sites from inactive ones
3. to predict further disease progression
4. to monitor the response to periodontal therapy (Buduneli and Kinane 2011) (Box 5.1).

Box 5.1 Expectations from the Biomarkers

Questions to be answered
• Who is susceptible/who is at risk?
• When is it active/is it progressing?
• Are there subtypes?

In an infectious and inflammatory chronic disease like periodontitis, there are three stages: infection, inflammation, and tissue destruction. Hence, the biomarker search may aim finding valid biomarkers identifying one or more of these

N. Buduneli, *Biomarkers in Periodontal Health and Disease*,
https://doi.org/10.1007/978-3-030-37317-7_5

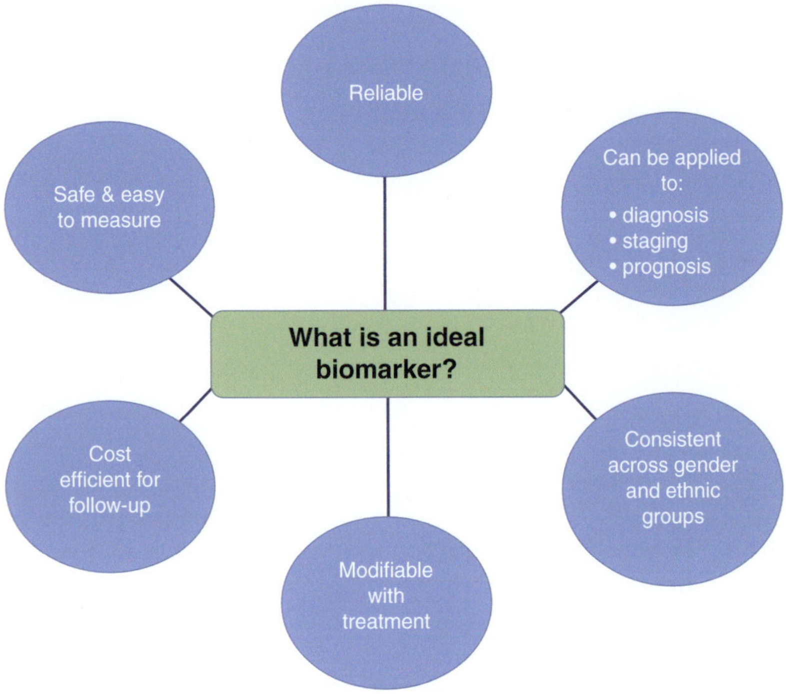

Fig. 5.1 Characteristics of an ideal biomarker for periodontal diseases

stages. Periodontal diseases have some unique characteristics as follows:

- They are very prevalent
- There are susceptibility/resistance; risk factors
- Infection, inflammation; focal infection theory is involved
- There are multifactorial/complex mechanisms
- There are unexplained cases

5.2 Microbial Factors for the Diagnosis of Periodontal Diseases

More than 700 bacterial species have been identified from subgingival plaque, but only a small number have been suggested to play a causal role in the pathogenesis of periodontal diseases (Socransky and Haffajee 2002). A number of specific periodontal pathogens have been implicated in periodontal diseases, including *Porphyromonas gingivalis, Tannerella forsythia,* and *Treponema denticola*. These are the members of the "red complex" and exhibit benzoyl-DL-arginine-naphthylamide, or BANA, activity (Loesche et al. 1992), and they are considered as putative periodontopathogens. The goal of microbiologic monitoring has been twofold; disease monitoring and guidance for treatment. However, BANA test, DNA probe analysis or culturing has failed to provide data predicting future disease progression. ELISA-based *Porphyromonas gingivalis* saliva kit can specifically detect this bacterium in saliva samples in just 90 s (O'Brien-Simpson et al. 2015). Compared with RT-PCR technology, the *Porphyromonas gingivalis* saliva kit is rapid and has a sensitivity of 92% and a specificity of 96%. A recent controlled clinical trial reported promising data about a newly developed chair-side test that can detect *Porphyromonas gingivalis, Tannerella forsythia, Treponema denticola, Prevotella intermedia,* and *Aggregatibacter actinomycetemcomitans* in sulcus fluid samples (Arweiler et al. 2019). It was stated that the chair-side test could detect these bacteria with a somewhat lower sensitivity compared to qPCR, but the detection sensitivity was classified as "good". There is a huge increase in recent knowledge on the ecology and microbiology of the oral cavity generated by "OMIC" Technologies and in the near future the knowledge can be clinically translated to support patient care, for prevention, monitoring, risk classification or early diagnosis of periodontal diseases. The suffix –ome is used to address the objects of study of fields, such as genome, proteome, or metabolome, respectively, and refers to a totality of some sort. OMICS aims at the collective characterisation and quantification of pools of biological molecules that translate into the structure, function, and dynamics of an organism of as many genes as possible of a given organism.

Analysis of saliva or GCF samples from periodontitis patients using proteolytic activity tests indicated that the presence of *Porphyromonas gingivalis* proteases is feasible (Kaman et al. 2012). Screening for the development of red plaque fluorescence may also have a diagnostic potential in the identification of high-risk individuals. Indeed, this feature of dental biofilm correlated with clinical periodontal diagnosis (van der Veen et al. 2016). Further longitudinal studies evaluating ecological changes in the oral cavity may explain the dysbiotic shift in the oral microbiome and provide valuable data not only for diagnosis but also for monitorisation of periodontitis (Tables 5.1 and 5.2).

5.3 Biomarkers for Detection of Periodontal Disease

Acute phase proteins include C-reactive protein (CRP), complement and coagulation factors, transport proteins, amyloid, and anti-protease enzymes. They are involved in positive or negative effects of acute and chronic inflammation, including chemotaxis, phagocytosis, antioxidant protection, and tissue repair. CRP, fibrinogen, and plasminogen-activator inhibitor have received much interest (Hajishengallis 2014; Lorenzo-Poso et al. 2018).

Gingival tissue and gingival crevicular fluid (GCF) concentrations of receptor activator of nuclear factor kappaB ligand (RANKL) and osteoprotegerin (OPG) have been investigated in numerous clinical human studies comparing periodontitis and healthy periodontium. The exact concentrations are variable among studies, but there is a clear trend indicating an increase in the RANKL/OPG ratio in periodontitis sites com-

Table 5.1 Microbiological and genetic tests commercially available

Biofluid	Target	Technique/product
Saliva	Detects type and concentration of bacteria	DNA PCR/my PerioPath®
Saliva	*P. intermedia, A.a, F. nucleatum, E. corrodens, C. rectus, T. forsythia, T. denticola*	DNA probe/OMNIgene®
	Trypsin-like protease (indirect detection of *P. gingivalis, T. denticola, T. forsythia,* and some *Capnocytophaga* strains)	Perioscan® (BANA test)
	P. gingivalis, P. intermedia, A.a.	Membrane-based enzyme immunoassay/Evalusite®
	Volatile sulphur compounds (indicates subgingival bacterial load)	Perioscan/Diamond probe/Perio 2000 system
	Bacterial toxins and protease (indicates disease activity by the change in the colour intensity scale)	Detects actively dividing and growing pathogens/TOPAS
Saliva	Determination of genetic susceptibility	MyperioID®

Table 5.2 Candidate biomarkers in saliva

Markers of soft tissue inflammation	Markers of alveolar bone loss	Collagen breakdown products
Prostaglandin E_2	Alkaline phosphatase	Aspartate aminotransferase
β-glucuronidase	Osteoprotegerin	Alanine aminotransferase
Interleukin-1β	Osteocalcin	Tissue inhibitors of matrix metalloproteinases
Interleukin-6	Collagen telopeptide	Matrix metalloproteinases
Tumour necrosis Factor-α	Carboxyterminal telopeptide pyridinoline cross-links of type I collagen	α2-macroglobulin
Matrix metalloproteinase-8,-9,-13	Receptor activator of nuclear factor kappaB	
	Osteonectin	

pared to the healthy sites and this ratio seems to correlate well with tissue inflammation and bone destruction (Crotti et al. 2003; Mogi et al. 2004; Wara-aswapati et al. 2007).

Possible biomarkers can be grouped as markers of inflammation; markers of connective tissue breakdown; and markers of bone loss. Beta-glucuronidase, CRP, interleukin (IL)-1, IL-6, macrophage inflammatory protein-1alpha (MIP-1α), and tumour necrosis factor (TNF) are involved in periodontal inflammation (Miller et al. 2010). There are complex interactions between host cells acting in the inflammatory and immune reactions and also their products (Fig. 5.2). Salivary levels of β-glucuronidase were found to be correlated with the severity of periodontitis (Lamster et al. 2003) and so were IL-1β levels (Tobon-Arroyave et al. 2008). IL-1 was previously known as osteoclast-activating factor and it is potent bone-resorbing cytokine produced primarily by activated macrophages, lymphocytes but also by fibroblasts, keratinocytes, endothelial cells, and mast cells. Bacterial LPS stimulates its secretion. IL-1β can be considered as one of the most common biomarkers that provide precise results as an indicator for periodontal disease progression (Ghallab 2018). IL-1β is initially released to fight with the infectious agents, however, when the infection extends, IL-1β initiates a cascade of events that leads to tissue destruction as is in case of periodontitis (Graves and Cochran 2013). IL-1β can be suggested as one of the most useful biomarkers for periodontal disease. TNF-α induces fibroblast apoptosis and leads a reduction in the repair capacity of periodontal tissues. Together with IL-6 and TNF-α GCF levels of IL-1β are increased in periodontitis sites and decrease the following successful treatment.

A more recent study investigating the newly discovered cytokine IL-35 exhibited the highest salivary level in the periodontally healthy group compared to the gingivitis and periodontitis groups and the authors concluded that the finding con-

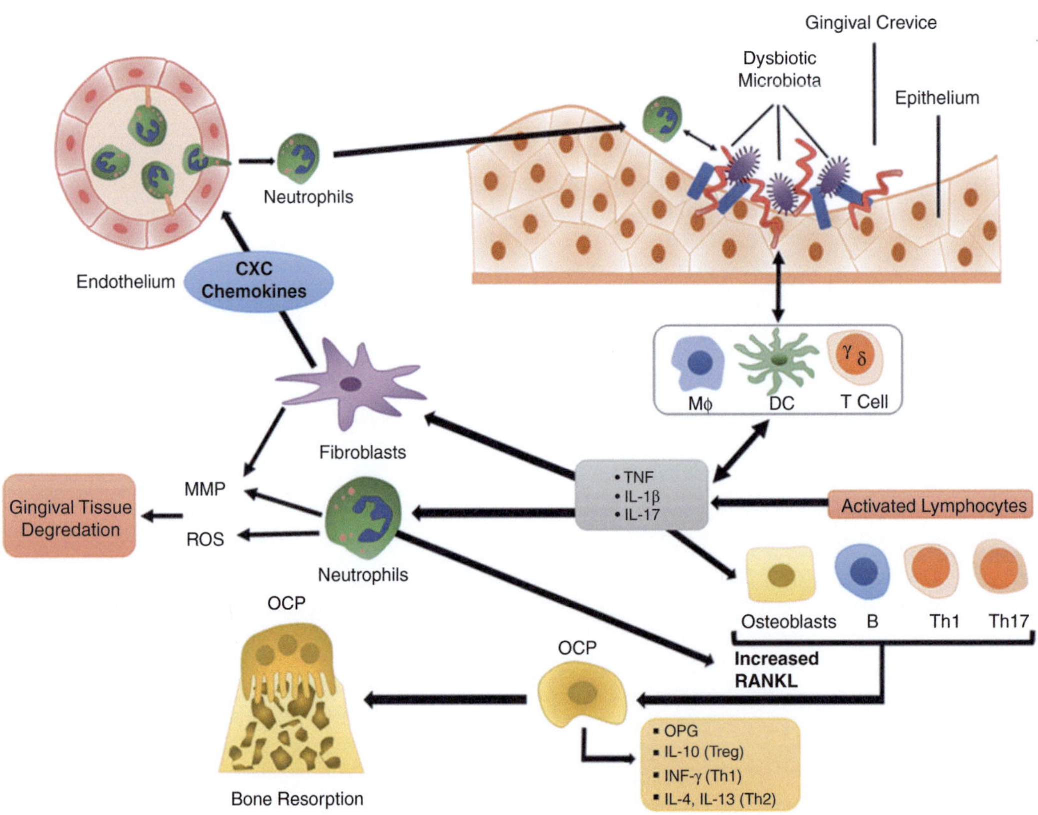

Fig. 5.2 Complex interactions between inflammatory cells and their products

firms the suppressive role of this cytokine on periodontal inflammation (Köseoğlu et al. 2015). Gümüş et al. (2017) investigated salivary and serum IL-33, IL-21, and prostaglandin E2 (PGE2) levels in generalised chronic or aggressive periodontitis patients and periodontally healthy individuals. The study provided further support for the role of IL-21 and IL-33 in periodontitis, but failed to detect discriminating role of these cytokines between aggressive and chronic periodontitis. This finding is in line with the 2017 classification that omitted this discrimination.

A recent systematic review and meta-analysis reported that only salivary levels of macrophage inflammatory protein-1a (MIP-1a) investigated by Al-Sabbagh et al. (2012) exhibited satisfactory results for all the test indicators required in an excellent test (de Lima et al. 2016). On the other hand, salivary biomarkers IL-6 and IL-1β evaluated by Ebersole et al. (2013) and Sanchez et al. (2013) showed acceptable values of diagnostic accuracy.

Monocyte chemoattractant protein-1 (MCP-1) is an important chemokine acting in the recruitment of inflammatory cells to the periodontal lesion. There are studies reporting increased GCF and salivary levels of MCP-1 and MCP-4 proportional to the progressing periodontitis severity as well as decreased levels with periodontal treatment (Gupta et al. 2013).

IL-8 is an important chemokine in periodontal diseases. It is released from endothelial cells, gingival fibroblasts, neutrophils, monocytes, and phagocytes in the gingival crevice and it is a potent chemoattractant of neutrophils. A recent study provided a systematic review of the available data on IL-8 mRNA and protein levels in gingival tissue, saliva, and GCF in patients with periodontitis (Finoti et al. 2017). The meta-analysis results demonstrated significantly lower levels of IL-8 in the GCF of patients with periodontitis. On the other hand, the majority of studies investigating gingival tissues found higher levels of IL-8 gene expression and IL-8 protein levels. The saliva data for IL-8 protein levels were inconclusive. It is likely that IL-8 can play multifunctional role in the pathogenesis of periodontitis, however, further studies are required to clarify its place.

Pentraxins are among the acute phase proteins and they function in the humoral arm of the innate immunity. They are a super family of multifunctional molecules that can be either short or long. Salivary levels of pentraxin3 (PTX3) were suggested to be related with periodontal inflammation (Gümüş et al. 2014a, b). Today, PTX3 is believed to be the true independent indicator of disease activity and may have clinical implication in diagnosing the sites at risk of losing attachment (Kathariya et al. 2013). B-lymphocytes play a central role in the adaptive immune response against invading pathogens in periodontitis. Cytokines, such as B-cell activating factor (BAFF), TNF-α, a proliferation-inducing ligand (APRIL), IL-6, and IL-10 that are important mediators of B-lymphocyte functions, were investigated in a cross-sectional study (Gümüş et al. 2014a, b). The authors concluded that elevated salivary and serum levels of TNF-a, APRIL, and BAFF may have a contributing role in the B-cell dominance in periodontitis.

Connective tissue breakdown is a critical step in progression from gingivitis to periodontitis. Locally produced proteases are responsible for the matrix degradation and most of these proteases are released by host cells, such as fibroblasts and neutrophils. Matrix metalloproteinases (MMPs) are produced in different forms, in latent, non-active pro-forms, and activated extra- or intracellularly depending on the structure of the MMP molecule (Nagase 1997). Among all MMPs, MMP-8, and -9 are associated with periodontal disease and neutrophil collagenase/MMP-8 is released by neutrophils, endothelial and smooth muscle cells, and macrophages upon inflammatory stimulus. MMP-8 is the protease that has been mostly investigated and its salivary and GCF levels correlate well with the severity of periodontitis (Marcaccini et al. 2010; Hernandez et al. 2012; Romero et al. 2013). Nizam et al. (2014) reported the elevated salivary and serum levels of neutrophil elastase (NE) and myeloperoxidase (MPO), lower levels of tissue inhibitor of MMP (TIMP)-1 in the periodontitis patients compared to the periodontally healthy control group supporting a close relationship between these proteases and clinical periodontal parameters in the generalised periodontitis patients. Type

I collagen comprises the majority of the organic component in periodontal matrix and therefore, collagenases are important in tissue destruction. MMP-8 is the main collagenase in periodontitis and 90–95% of collagenolytic activity in GCF originates from MMP-8. This enzyme can degrade type I and III collagen (Franco et al. 2017). A recent study provided a systematic review and meta-analysis on the diagnostic role of salivary MMP-8 levels (Zhang et al. 2018). The salivary MMP-8 level varied greatly between different studies, which vary in terms of salivary flow rate, use of antimicrobial agents, and also smoking habits of the participants. Different detection methods like ELISA, IFMA, and Luminex may also influence the data variation. The salivary MMP-8 levels were significantly higher in periodontitis patients than those in healthy controls. However, the great variation observed in the meta-analysis does not enable making a strong conclusion and prospective, large-scale studies with well-defined patient characteristics are required to better clarify the potential of MMP-8 as a diagnostic biomarker for periodontitis. On the other hand, the Helsinki group developed a point-of-care diagnostic test evaluating salivary MMP-8 levels (PerioSafe®, ImplantSafe®). These tests depend on the lateral flow chromatography, claimed to identify and screen chronic and initial periodontitis sites and patients, differentiate active sites and patients, predict disease progression, and can be utilised to monitoring the treatment and medication as well as during the maintenance (Leppilahti et al. 2014a, b; Heikkenen et al. 2016). Moreover, it is supposed to identify genetically predisposed adolescents (Heikkenen et al. 2017). The test sticks can be quantitated by the ORALyser reader in 5 min PoC/chair-side. A positive aMMP-8 test is based on a cut-off of 25 ng aMMP-8 per millilitre or filtrate derived from 5 mL mouth rinse. The sensitivity and specificity of the aMMP-8 test have been demonstrated to be 76.5% and 96.7% for >2 sites and deepened pockets, respectively (Rathnayake et al. 2017). The MMP-8 dip-stick-test also agreed very well with quantitative laboratory immunofluorescence assay (IFMA) and showed specificity of 0.96 and sensitivity of 0.83 (Mantyla et al. 2003).

Numerous studies have been published investigating possible biomarkers for alveolar bone loss in periodontitis. The episodic nature of periodontitis is one of the difficulties in the identification of clear biomarkers and longitudinal studies are required for monitoring stable and progressing periodontitis cases either patient-based or site-based. However, such longitudinal and powered studies are highly costly. The salivary levels of candidate biomarkers are usually very low and depending on the laboratory detection technique, may be below the detection limit (Frodge et al. 2008). Alkaline phosphatase (ALP), carboxyterminal telopeptide pyridinoline cross-links of type I collagen (ICTP), RANKL, OPG are among the most possible biomarkers for bone destruction in periodontitis. Periodontitis patients exhibited significantly lower plasma concentrations of OPG and an increased ratio of RANKL/OPG possibly having a role in the susceptibility of these patients for periodontitis (Özçaka et al. 2010). GCF levels of OPG were significantly lower and those of IL-1β, sRANKL together with the sRANKL/OPG ratio were significantly higher in periodontitis sites compared to the periodontally healthy sites (Gürlek et al. 2017).

GCF pyridinoline cross-linked carboxyterminal telopeptide of type I collagen has been reported to be a good biomarker for future alveolar bone and attachment loss also well correlating with clinical parameters and putative periodontal pathogens (Giannobile 1999).

Reactive oxygen species (ROS), when produces in excessive amounts may cause oxidative stress. ROS is most closely related to neutrophil actions in the destruction of periodontal pathogens. Increased ROS levels may cause tissue damage and worsen the periodontal disease. Antioxidants are produced by various cells to balance the effects of reactive oxygen species, free radicals, and other reactive molecular species. One of the most important markers of oxidative stress is 8-hydroxy-2-deoxyguanosine (8-OHdG), which is formed through the oxidation of guanine from damaged DNA (Buczko et al. 2015). A recent meta-analysis reported that salivary 8-OHdG levels in patients with periodontal disease were 2.11 ng/ml higher than those of the healthy controls, almost doubling the concentration in periodontally healthy individuals and the salivary level of this antioxidant was suggested as a powerful biomarker for periodontal disease (Paredes-Sanchez et al. 2018).

In general, any deviation from normal neutrophil activity (diminished or excessive recruitment; impaired function or hyperactivity) causes disruption of periodontal tissue homeostasis leading to periodontitis (Ryder 2010; Hajishengallis and Hajishengallis 2014). Neutrophils can cause periodontal tissue destruction through the release of degradative enzymes such as MMPs or cytotoxic substances such as reactive oxygen species (Ryder 2010; Nussbaum and Shapira 2011). Neutrophils can also induce osteoclastic alveolar bone resorption through expression of membrane-bound RANKL as long as they are in close proximity to the bone (Chakravarti et al. 2009). Moreover, neutrophils can mediate indirect tissue destruction by chemotactic recruitment of IL-17 producing cells (Pelletier et al. 2010) (Fig. 5.3).

Th1 cells are primarily responsible for cell mediated immunity to intracellular pathogens (bacteria, protozoa, and viruses) and have been implicated in inflammatory diseases. Th2 cells, on the other hand, mediate humoral immunity including the production of IgE. The recently described Th17 subset mediates responses reinforcing neutrophil and innate immunity functions. TGF-β, IL-6, IL-1 are important for the differentiation of Th17. Th1 cells predominate the stable lesions, whereas Th2 cells are associated with progression of periodontitis that means progressing lesions are rich in B-cells and plasma cells (Gemmell et al. 2007).

IL-17 family of cytokines consists of IL-17A, IL-17B, IL-17C, IL-17D, IL-17E (IL-25), and IL-17F. IL-17A synergizes with other cytokines, including IL-1β, TNF-α (Korn et al. 2009). IL-17A can potentially induce the expression of MMPs in fibroblasts, endothelial cells, and epithelial cells as well as increasing RANKL expression and concomitantly decreases OPG

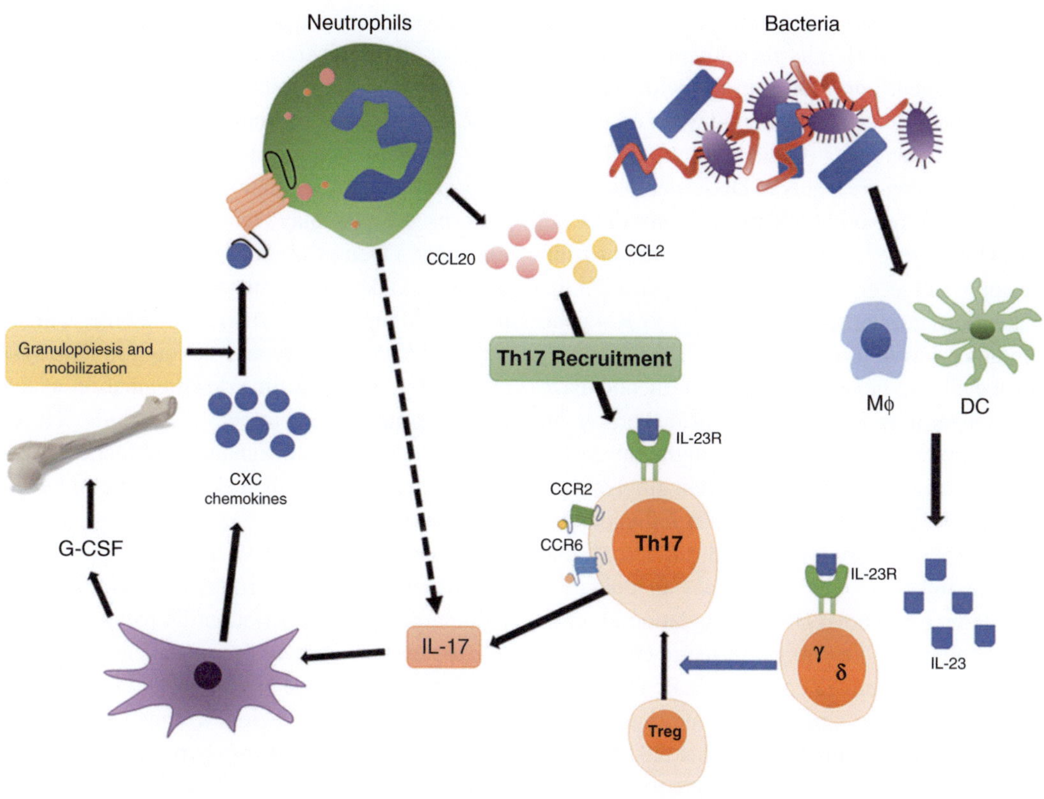

Fig. 5.3 IL-17 cytokines in the interaction between neutrophils and bacteria

expression in osteoblastic cells in vitro and in vivo (Lester et al. 2007). Hence, IL-17 can mediate destruction of both connective tissue and the underlying bone. IL-17F also plays a critical role in host defence upon bacterial and fungal infection by recruiting neutrophils and producing antimicrobial-peptides (Iwakura et al. 2008). The presence of IL-17A/F heterodimers substantially influences the potency, specificity and the spectrum of the activity of cytokines (Chang and Dong 2007). In contrast with the other IL-17 family cytokines, IL-17E is an anti-inflammatory cytokine, which opposes the functions of IL-17A and IL-17F (Monteleone et al. 2010). Salivary and plasma levels of IL-17 and IL-18 were compared between chronic periodontitis patients and periodontally healthy individuals and salivary IL-18 level was suggested as a possible biomarker for periodontitis (Özçaka et al. 2011).

Epigenetics of periodontal disease has attracted great interest with several observations both at the level of DNA and histone proteins. Gingival tissues from periodontitis patients have altered epigenetic patterns, particularly at inflammation-related genes (Barros and Offenbacher 2014). The methylation pattern of the IL-8 gene promoter in individuals with chronic periodontitis was altered when compared with healthy subjects (Oliveira et al. 2009). In a study analysing the status of DNA methylation in the promoter region of toll-like receptor (TLR)-2 and TLR-4 genes in gingival tissue samples from healthy subjects and chronic periodontitis patients, major unmethylation of the TLR-4 gene promoter was found in all groups, but the results for the TLR-2 gene promoter were inconclusive (De Oliveira et al. 2011). Benakanakere et al. (2015) noted sporadic DNA methylation on the promoter region of TLR-2 in certain gingival epithelial cells that exhibited blunted inflammatory responses to *P. gingivalis* and suggested that chronic infection of *P. gingivalis* in epithelial cells induced de novo DNA methylation in vitro. Wide epigenetic alterations in many chemokine and cytokine genes in epithelial cells from periodontitis affected gingival tissue have been reported (Barros and Offenbacher 2014). It is plausible that the differences in epigenetic signatures on pattern recognition receptors may help explain periodontitis disease susceptibility (Benakanakere et al. 2015).

TLRs play a pivotal role in periodontitis and abnormal expression of TLRs can be observed in subjects with periodontitis. LPS signalling is mediated by TLRs leading to NFkB activation. Saliva can serve as a diagnostic fluid in periodontitis (Sahingur and Cohen 2004). Reduced salivary soluble TLR-2 levels were found in periodontitis patients that were increased following successful periodontal treatment (Prakasam and Srinivasan 2014). Salivary TLR-4 levels were found to be elevated in periodontitis patients compared to the periodontally healthy controls (Buduneli et al. 2011). Moreover, TLR-2 and TLR-4 levels in plasma of the same periodontitis patients were higher than the healthy controls. The current literature indicates a trend for upregulation of TLRs in periodontitis patients and therefore, they have the potential to serve as diagnostic or prognostic biomarkers for periodontitis.

A typical inflammatory response results in the upregulation of genes associated with the production of lectins that then coat epithelial cell surfaces, with the function of recruiting neutrophils to the site of inflammation (Lindroth and Park, 2013). Then an immune response is initiated comprising both innate and acquired systems. Epigenetic regulation of gene expression patterns seems to play the most important role at this stage (Wen et al. 2008). Epigenetic mechanisms also take the key step in the upregulation of the pro-inflammatory cytokines and other signalling molecules to fully activate the immune system, and at the same time downregulation of the anti-inflammatory cytokines (Tsuchida et al. 2019). Inflammation signalling influences epigenetic changes in cells making the picture even more complex.

Gingival epithelial cells have a unique capacity to respond to environmental factors. The inflamed gingiva in periodontitis patients shows overexpression of cytokines, such as IL-6 and interferon-gamma (IFN-γ) (Babel et al. 2006; Zhang et al. 2010). There are evidences for epigenetic changes related with hypermethylation of TNF-α promoter, IFN-γ, and COX-2 enzyme (Zhang et al. 2010, 2013; Loo et al. 2010).

MicroRNAs (miRNAs) are small, endogenous, non-coding RNAs approximately 20–22 nucleotides in length. They act in a sequence-specific manner and regulate gene expression at the post-transcriptional level through cleavage or translational repression of their target mRNAs (Kagiya 2015). miRNAs are now accepted to be involved in periodontal tissue homeostasis and most of them are likely to be related with osteoclast differentiation (Kagiya 2016). mir-21 is highly expressed in gingiva in periodontitis and also in cells during osteoclastogenesis. It is yet not clarified whether miRNAs exist in GCF, but it is likely that future studies will provide the evidence for their usage as biomarkers of periodontal disease. Saliva and serum are more likely to be the source biofluids. There are limited studies investigating the potential of miRNAs as diagnostic biomarkers in periodontal diseases and there are severe variations in their methodologies disabling to make a clear conclusion. Further studies with standardised methodology are warranted to better clarify the issue.

5.4 Biomarkers for Prognosis of Non-surgical Periodontal Treatment

Periodontitis is a chronic infectious disease that is characterised by persistent inflammation, connective tissue breakdown, and alveolar bone destruction (Armitage 1999). It was reported to be the sixth most prevalent chronic inflammatory disease in the world with an overall prevalence of 11.2% (Kassebaum et al. 2014). The prevalence of periodontitis increases with age (Eke et al. 2012). Microbial dental plaque is the initiating factor for periodontal diseases and various local, systemic and environmental factors modify the disease progression (Kinane et al. 2006). More than 700 different microorganism species have been detected in the oral cavity (Aas et al. 2005), and more than 400 species can be found in subgingival plaque samples (Paster et al. 2001). It is accepted that the clinical findings of periodontal disease are the result of the complex interactions between the host and bacteria.

Clinical periodontal diagnosis relies mainly on evaluation of gingival inflammation, level of oral hygiene, and visual signs of periodontal tissue destruction. Classical parameters include measurement of probing depth (PD), clinical attachment level (CAL), plaque index (PI), bleeding on probing (BOP), and radiographic findings. Accurate diagnosis at the patient level requires full mouth clinical measurements by a periodontal probe at four/six sites per tooth, which is quite laborious. Moreover, the accuracy of these clinical measurements is affected by various internal and external factors, such as the degree of inflammation, anatomical factors of the dentition, experience of the clinician, design of the periodontal probe, etc. Although these clinical parameters are the best currently available indicators for determining disease status they only reflect the past periodontal tissue destruction and provide little or no information on the current disease activity nor predict future activity (Haffajee et al. 1983). Their specificity and sensitivity are low. Therefore, novel diagnostic and monitoring methods are highly desired for screening of susceptibility, diagnosing periodontal disease, evaluating the response to treatment, and predicting future tissue destruction. A vast number of studies have focused on defining biomarkers for periodontal diagnosis and monitoring purposes.

Accordingly, it would be highly desirable to develop reliable, innovative, simple, and non-invasive diagnostic methods for early detection of active disease and for monitoring the response to periodontal treatment (Giannobile et al. 2009). The clinical value of a diagnostics test relies on the answers to the questions below (Mombelli 2005):

- Does the test provide truly new information?
- Is there a treatment alternative?
- Is it less expensive to treat than to test?
- What are the unwanted effects of an intervention?
- What are the consequences of no treatment?

A biomarker is described as an objective indication of the medical state observed from outside the patient—which can be measured accurately and reproducibly. It is measurable, it can act as a reliable indicator of the biological process and it can be applied to diagnosis, staging, and also prognosis of a certain disease. An ideal biomarker should be relevant and valid. Furthermore, it should be safe and easy to measure, modifiable with treatment, thus reflecting the response to treatment. It should also be cost-efficient to follow-up and consistent across gender and different ethnic groups. Apart from these prerequisites, a real biomarker has to be beneficial in clinical practice rather than just confirming a clinically established diagnosis. A true biomarker can serve as the diagnostic tool and enlighten the path to the accurate clinical diagnosis or even the treatment plan in the absence of a periodontist. This may sound a little bit unrealistic or utopic, but such circumstances may already exist.

The ideal diagnostic test should have high sensitivity, specificity, and predictive value. Sensitivity relates to the test's intrinsic ability to correctly detect patients who have a disease. Specificity relates to the test's intrinsic ability to correctly detect patients without a disease. The positive and negative predictive values are the proportions of positive and negative results in diagnostic tests that are true positive and true negative. They describe the performance of a diagnostic test, and are not only intrinsic to the test but also depend on the prevalence of the disease.

Several molecules including enzymes, cytokines, receptors, and other proteins have been studied as potential biomarkers for periodontal diseases. These biomarkers can be found in various biofluids, such as gingival crevicular fluid (GCF); blood, serum or plasma; and saliva. GCF has the advantage of providing information at the site level, but its collection is time-consuming, requires special instruments and experienced personnel and the sample's volume is very low. On the other hand, large volumes of saliva samples can be obtained easily. Its collection procedure is fast, non-invasive, and more convenient for both the patient and the clinician. However, saliva cannot provide site-specific information as it contains local and systemic markers of periodontal disease (Kaufman and Lamster 2000). Accordingly, blood cannot provide site-specific information and its sampling is invasive compared to that of saliva. However, it can be collected easily and does not require a dental office. Due to this simple, fast, and relatively non-invasive method of collection together with the ability of reflecting systemic health state, salivary and blood diagnostic tests are promising for diagnosis and monitoring of periodontal disease at the patient level.

5.5 Biomarkers for Monitoring of Disease Progress

Various cytokines, enzymes, or molecules in blood or saliva have been studied for their potential to be utilised for monitoring the response to periodontal treatment. Among the most studied biomarkers are; serum high sensitive C-reactive protein (hsCRP), interleukin-6 (IL-6), oncostatin M, matrix metalloproteinase-8 (MMP-8) and MMP-9, and salivary sCD44, arginase, soluble RANKL (sRANKL), and OPG.

5.5.1 Response to Treatment

Non-surgical periodontal treatment is the first and mandatory step of the periodontal treatment in each and every patient with some sort of periodontal disease. It comprises patient motivation and instruction on better oral hygiene, scaling and root planing, and removal of plaque retentive factors such as overhanging restorations from the mouth. Periodontitis patients need to be re-evaluated 2–3 months after the completion of non-surgical periodontal treatment. At this stage, the clinician decides whether additional treatment modalities such as administration of antimicrobials or surgical periodontal treatment are required to improve the treatment outcomes.

Early diagnosis of periodontal disease may provide benefits as follows:

- developing individually tailored treatment modalities,
- improving quality of life,

- preserving masticatory function,
- decreasing lifelong financial burden.

In a comprehensive study, Behle et al. (2009) investigated 19 inflammatory biomarkers in patients with chronic periodontitis before and after non-surgical and also surgical periodontal treatment. They reported high individual variability and poor correlation between inflammatory markers and clinical, microbiological, and serological markers of periodontitis (Behle et al. 2009). On the other hand, significant decreases in serum high sensitivity C reactive protein (hsCRP) and IL-6 during the first 3 months after scaling and root planing have been reported and these changes correlated with the improvement in clinical periodontal parameters (Marcaccini et al. 2009a, Nakajima et al. 2010). Furthermore, anti-inflammatory therapy with chemical agents alone has been shown to significantly decrease serum concentrations of hsCRP, IL-6, and interferon (IFN) in patients with periodontitis (Renvert et al. 2009). However, the authors failed to detect any significant improvement in clinical parameters without mechanical periodontal therapy. In a multi-centre study, Offenbacher et al. (2009) reported that serum hsCRP levels were similar in patients receiving scaling and root planing and those patients receiving community care. However, there was a great variability in terms of the treatment provided in community care, and obesity was a confounding factor that nullified the periodontal treatment effects on hsCRP reduction (Offenbacher et al. 2009). Available data suggest that serum hsCRP and IL-6 are promising systemic biomarkers for monitoring the response to periodontal treatment in systemically healthy, non-smoker, non-obese patients who do not take any anti-inflammatory medications.

In another intervention study, Duarte et al. (2010) comparatively evaluated the serum concentration of several cytokines in patients with generalised chronic periodontitis, generalised aggressive periodontitis and healthy controls, and the effect of periodontal therapy on these cytokines 6 months after the completion of periodontal treatment. Tumour necrosis factor-alpha (TNF-α) and IL-17 concentrations were significantly higher in the aggressive periodontitis patients compared to the healthy controls or patients with chronic periodontitis, while there was no difference in other cytokines (Duarte et al. 2010). Furthermore, non-surgical periodontal therapy significantly decreased plasma TNF-α and IL-17 concentrations compared to the baseline values; both results were statistically significant, however, TNF-α levels remained elevated compared to healthy controls. These results suggest that serum TNF-α and IL-17 may be useful biomarkers for the differential diagnosis between aggressive and chronic periodontitis, while IL-17 may be more helpful for monitoring the response to periodontal treatment in the aggressive periodontitis patients. These studies have lost their place to some extent; there is no more differentiation between aggressive and chronic periodontitis forms as after the 2017 classification.

Oncostatin M, a member of the IL-6 family of cytokines, is synthesised and secreted by T-cells and monocytes in response to bacterial products; it has been shown to have a key role in regulating periodontal bone resorption, by acting on both osteoblast and osteoclast receptor RANKL regulation (Lu et al. 2006). Serum oncostatin M concentration was significantly higher in patients with chronic periodontitis compared to patients with gingivitis or periodontally healthy controls (Pradeep et al. 2010). Furthermore, oncostatin M concentration decreased significantly 2 months after the completion of non-surgical periodontal therapy, and this decrease positively correlated with the improvement in clinical periodontal parameters. These data suggest that serum oncostatin M may be a useful biomarker for the diagnosis as well as monitoring the response to periodontal treatment.

Marcaccini et al. (2009b) evaluated the plasma concentrations of several matrix metalloproteinases (MMPs) and tissue inhibitors of MMPs (TIMPs) in patients with chronic periodontitis and also healthy controls, and the effect of periodontal therapy on these enzymes 3 months after the completion of periodontal treatment. They found that MMP-3, MMP-8, and MMP-9 concentrations were significantly higher in periodontitis patients compared with healthy controls, while there was no difference in MMP-2, TIMP-1, and TIMP-2 levels. Furthermore, non-surgical periodontal therapy significantly reduced plasma MMP-8 and MMP-9 concentrations compared to the baseline values. These results suggest that plasma MMP-3, −8, and − 9 may be useful biomarkers for the diagnosis of diseased individuals, while MMP-8 and -9 may be useful for monitoring response to periodontal treatment.

RANK is found on the surface of osteoclasts; along with its agonist, RANKL, and its antagonist, OPG, they are the three key molecules for coordinating osteoclastogenesis and alveolar bone resorption (Suda et al. 1999). RANKL and OPG have been studied mainly in GCF samples and their concentrations show a great variation between different studies. In a cross-sectional study, Buduneli et al. (2008) found that salivary RANKL levels were significantly lower in non-smoker patients in the maintenance phase compared to the untreated non-smoker patients. When comparing smokers in the maintenance phase to untreated smokers, this difference was not significant, indicating that smoking affects RANKL and OPG levels and prevents their being biomarkers to determine disease status in smokers. This data suggest that salivary RANKL may be a promising systemic biomarker for monitoring response to periodontal treatment in non-smokers but not in smokers.

CD44 is a cell-surface adhesion molecule that is known to mediate cell–cell and cell–matrix interactions, and support cell migration, including neutrophil adhesion and transendothelial migration (Khan et al. 2004; Zhuo et al. 2006). In a pilot intervention study evaluating the effect of scaling and root planing on salivary sCD44 levels, Ghallab and Shaker (2010) found that treatment resulted in significant decrease in sCD44 in patients with chronic periodontitis at 1 month after treatment. Furthermore, this decrease was observed in both smokers and non-smokers, suggesting that salivary sCD44 may be a promising systemic biomarker for monitoring response to periodontal treatment in both smokers and non-smokers.

Endocan is a proteoglycan secreted by endothelial cells under the control of inflammatory cytokines (Bechard et al. 2000). Vascular endothelial growth factor (VEGF-A) is derived from platelets and plays an important role in endothelial cell proliferation, proteolytic enzyme secretion, and migration through chemotaxis; it also stimulates angiogenesis (Shibuya 2013). Possible effects of non-surgical periodontal treatment on serum and GCF levels of endocan, TNF-α, and VEGF-A have been investigated in a group of generalised chronic periodontitis patients (Türer et al. 2017). Biofluid samples were obtained at baseline and then 6 weeks after the completion of non-surgical periodontal treatment. The authors reported higher biomarker levels in periodontitis patients compared to the healthy controls and these levels decreased significantly after periodontal treatment. Therefore, endocan was suggested to be a candidate diagnostic and prognostic biomarker.

Arginase is the final enzyme in the urea cycle that converts L-arginine to urea and L-ornithine, and, although it is mainly found in the human liver, it is also present in some extrahepatic tissues, including salivary glands. Nitric oxide is a free radical with antimicrobial activity that has been shown to be produced in response to periodontal pathogens (Akopov and Kankanian 1996). Nitric oxide is produced by L-arginine under the action of an isoenzyme called NOS. Gheren et al. (2008) compared the salivary arginase activity in patients with chronic periodontitis and healthy controls, and also evaluated the effect of periodontal therapy on the activity of this enzyme 1 month after periodontal treatment. Salivary arginase activity was 2.5 times higher in the chronic periodontitis patients when compared to periodontally healthy controls, and periodontal therapy significantly reduced salivary arginase activity levels. Salivary arginase activity positively correlated with clinical periodontal parameters and could distinguish periodontitis patients and controls, but there was no significant correlation between salivary arginase activity level and severity of periodontitis. These results suggest that salivary arginase activity may be a useful biomarker for the diagnosis of diseased individuals, but it does not seem to be helpful for determining disease severity or for monitoring response to periodontal treatment.

Aspartate aminotransferase (AST), alanine aminotransferase (ALT), and lactate dehydrogenase (LDH) are intracellular enzymes released from the damaged cells of periodontal tissues into the GCF and saliva. Yoshie et al. (2007) found that non-surgical periodontal treatment reduced LDH levels in all patients with chronic periodontitis. All results for all enzymes were consistent between smokers and non-smokers. This data suggest that salivary LDH may be a promising systemic biomarker for monitoring response to periodontal treatment, and it is independent of smoking status.

In a recent study, Gul et al. (2017) assessed the ability of a novel combination of biomarkers to predict treatment outcome of patients with chronic periodontitis. The researchers collected GCF samples from 77 patients at baseline and also three, and 6 months after completion of non-surgical periodontal treatment. It was reported that using baseline values of MMP-8, elastase, and sialidase it could be possible to differentiate healthy from diseased sites. Furthermore, these biomarkers at baseline provided accurate predictions of treatment outcome on a site-specific basis.

Evaluating cumulative effects of bacterial and host-derived salivary biomarkers may be more accurate as diagnostic tools for periodontal disease. Indeed, the greatest diagnostic accuracy was found when the detection of the host biomarkers was coupled with those of the red complex periodontal pathogens (Ramseier et al. 2009).

5.6 Point-of-Care Diagnostics

Point-of-care tests are those developed to be used either chair-side by the clinician or at home by the patient. Home-used pregnancy test is an excellent example of such tests as it is simple, reliable, affordable, and fast (Loos and Tjoa 2005). Lab-on-a-chip and microfluidic devices are promising for particularly saliva and GCF samples. Such tests may also help to reveal episodes of disease activity in chronic periodontitis that has an episodic character (Giannobile et al. 2009) (Table 5.3).

5.7 Limitations of Available Studies

There are some major limitations of the studies aiming to identify diagnostic or prognostic biomarkers for periodontal diseases. First of all, the candidate biomarkers are correlated with clinical periodontal parameters mainly probing depth and clinical attachment level. Relying on solely clinical attachment level may lead to many false-positive diagnoses particularly in young study populations, whereas using solely probing depth may cause many false-negatives particularly in the older study populations. Whether or not these clinical measurements provide accurate information indirectly affects the accuracy of the biomarkers. Furthermore, there are great discrepancies in the

Table 5.3 Commercially available biochemical point-of-care (POC) diagnostics using saliva or GCF samples

Test kits	Functions	Target/diagnostic aim
Oral fluid nanosensor test	Detection of multiple salivary proteins and nucleic acids	Oral cancer (OFNASET)®
Electronic taste chips	Simultaneously monitor several biomarkers related to periodontal disease	Electronic tastechip (ETC): Can detect CRP at very low concentrations
OraQuick®	Fast and accurate test results in 20 min	Usually detects HIV 1 and HIV 2
Integrated microfluidic platform for oral diagnostics (IMPOD)®	Quantification of an oral disease biomarker	Can quantify MMP-8 and others in just 3–10 min
Periogard®	Detects aspartate aminotransferase (AST)	GCF AST level
Pocket watch®	Detects AST	GCF AST level
Periocheck®	Detects collagenase (neutral protease)	
Prognostic® (Dentisply), Biolise	Elastase (serine protease)	
PerioSafe®	Patient-based test	Detects salivary MMP-8
ImplantSafe®	Site-based test	Detects MMP-8 in GCF

clinical diagnostic criteria used in different studies and these differences also affect the conclusion about the biomarkers. Cross-sectional studies suffer from the risk of sampling stable state. Moreover, the methodological differences between different studies disable combining data from different sources. There is a great heterogeneity in patient/site inclusion criteria, blinding and calibration of the investigators, sampling technique, sample storage conditions, laboratory analysis method, statistical analysis, and data handling/reporting. Patient demographics as well as smoking status may well have an influence on the biochemical data.

Problems with papers:

- may not be powered
- publication bias exist; negative results are rarely published
- smoking status is not reported
- exclusion of smokers leads loss of data
- heterogeneous in methodology
- variety in data reporting

If you do not know where you are heading, it does not matter which way you go… Carol Lewis (Alis in Wonderland).

5.8 Conclusion

Approximately, a hundred different molecules have been investigated in GCF samples and some reports are controversial. Hence, not all assayed molecules seem to be promising as biomarkers for periodontal disease. The majority of candidate biomarkers in GCF and saliva are the indicators of inflammatory events that precede alveolar bone destruction. Current literature about the most studied markers that seem to be most relevant are provided here. Single candidate proteins have been extensively investigated by immunoassays in an attempt to find diagnostic and/or prognostic biomarkers for periodontal diseases. However, it became quite clear that a single marker would not be sufficient to fulfil the expectations. Moreover, it is highly likely that complex interactions among the host-derived and/or bacteria-derived factors play some critical roles in the phenotype of periodontal disease. Thus, researchers have headed towards investigating a combination of candidate markers either biochemical or microbiological. Today, a panel of markers is regarded to be more likely to provide strong information in addition to the clinical periodontal findings.

Systemic periodontal diagnostic tests are still at an early stage of development and much work is needed to validate their utility as an important and cost-effective aspect of clinical diagnosis, treatment planning, or patient monitoring. The diagnosis of periodontitis and also the most reliable prognostic indicators are currently based almost entirely on clinical periodontal measurements. However, these clinical measurements not only demonstrate low sensitivity and specificity as diagnostic tests, but also are subjective, laborious, and require a lot of chair time. In the past 30 years numerous studies have been undertaken in an attempt to find a point-of-care test that can reliably identify sites with actively progressing periodontitis. Pathogenic mechanisms involved in progression of periodontal tissue destruction are mainly related with the inflammatory and immune system. Multiple local and systemic periodontal diagnostic biomarkers have been proposed within the literature, however; there are still no tests that can detect active periodontal lesions during, or before, the episodes of progression. One major barrier is the fact that progressing and nonprogressing sites share a lot of features and this makes it a big challenge. The episodic character of progression, the multiple factors that are either host- or microorganism-related, the wide range of individual variability in the response to the microbial attacks and therapeutic measures are challenging for biomarker identification. Moreover, there is a great diversity between the studies in biological sample collection, storage, laboratory and statistical analyses methods, and data presentation. We still have some steps to take until we reach a breakthrough in the field of diagnostic tests for discrimination of active sites.

Large-scale and preferentially prospective studies investigating multiprotein complexes with/without microbiological parameters may provide the demanded answers in the near future. It is also imperative that future studies will strictly base the clinical diagnosis on the 2017 classification of periodontal diseases.

Key issues for future studies:

- candidate biomarkers should be validated with large populations
- clinical diagnostic criteria should be standardised
- saliva sampling method should be standardised
- detection methods should be comparable
- examiners should be calibrated
- studies should be preferentially longitudinal
- tests should be cost-effective
- statistical tests should be appropriate, comparable
- ELISA kits should be validated for the particular biofluids; saliva or GCF

No wind serves him, who addresses his voyage to no certain port! Montaigne.

References

Aas JA, Paster BJ, Stokes LN, Olsen I, Dewhirst FE. Defining the normal bacterial flora of the oral cavity. J Clin Microbiol. 2005;43:5721–32.

Akopov SE, Kankanian AP. Nitric oxide (NO) inactivation by polymorphonuclear leukocytes as a mechanism for the development of periodontal lesions. Stomatologiia (Mosk). 1996;75:12–4.

Al-Sabbagh M, Alladah A, Lin Y, Kryscio RJ, Thomas MV, Ebersole JL, Miller CS. Bone remodelling-associated salivary biomarker MIP-1alpha distinguishes periodontal disease from health. J Periodontal Res. 2012;47:389–95.

Armitage GC. Development of a classification system for periodontal diseases and conditions. Ann Periodontol. 1999;4:1–6.

Arweiler NB, Marx VK, Laugisch O, Sculean A, Auschill TM. Clinical evaluation of a newly developed chair side test to determine periodontal pathogens. J Periodontol. 2019. https://doi.org/10.1002/JPER.19-0180.

Babel N, Cherepnev G, Babel D, Tropmann A, Hammer M, Volk HD, et al. Analysis of tumour necrosis factor-alpha, transforming growth factor-beta, interleukin-10, IL-6, and interferon-gamma gene polymorphisms in patients with chronic periodontitis. J Periodontol. 2006;77:1978–83.

Barros SP, Offenbacher S. Modifiable risk factors in periodontal disease: epigenetic regulation of gene expression in the inflammatory response. Periodontol 2000. 2014;64:95–110.

Bechard D, Meignin V, Scherpereel A, et al. Characterization of the secreted form of endothelial-cell-specific molecule 1 by specific monoclonal antibodies. J Vasc Res. 2000;37:417–25.

Behle JH, Sedaghatfar MH, Demmer RT, et al. Heterogeneity of systemic inflammatory responses to periodontal therapy. J Clin Periodontol. 2009;36:287–94.

Benakanakere M, Abdolhosseini M, Hosur K, Finoti LS, Kinane DF. TLR2 promoter hypermethylation creates innate immune dysbiosis. J Dent Res. 2015;94:183–91.

Buczko P, Zalewska A, Szarmach I. Saliva and oxidative stress in oral cavity and in some systemic disorders. J Physiol Pharmacol. 2015;66:3–9.

Buduneli N, Kinane DF. Host-derived diagnostic markers related to soft tissue destruction and bone degradation in periodontitis. J Clin Periodontol. 2011;38(Suppl. 11):85–105.

Buduneli N, Bıyıkoğlu B, Sherrabeh S, Lappin DF. Saliva concentrations of RANKL and osteoprotegerin in smoker versus non-smoker chronic periodontitis patients. J Clin Periodontol. 2008;35:846–52.

Buduneli N, Ozcaka O, Nalbantsoy A. Salivary and plasma levels of toll-like receptor 2 and toll-like receptor 4 in chronic periodontitis. J Periodontol. 2011;82:878–84.

Chakravarti A, Raquil MA, Tessier P, Poubelle PE. Surface RANKL of toll-like receptor 4-stimulated human neutrophils activates osteoclastic bone resorption. Blood. 2009;114:1633–44.

Chang SH, Dong C. A novel heterodimeric cuyokine consisting of IL-17 and IL-17F regulates inflammatory response. Cell Res. 2007;17:435–40.

Crotti T, Smith MD, Hirsch R, et al. Receptor activator NF kappaB ligand (RANKL) and osteoprotegerin (OPG) protein expression in periodontitis. J Periodontal Res. 2003;38:380–7.

Curtis MA, Gillett IR, Griffiths GS, Maiden MF, Sterne JA, Wilson DT, et al. Detection of high-risk groups and individuals for periodontal diseases: laboratory markers from analysis of gingival crevicular fluid. J Clin Periodontol. 1989;16:1–11.

de Lima CL, Acevedo AC, Grisi DC, Taba Jr M, Guerra E, de Luca Canto G. Host-derived salivary biomarkers in diagnosing periodontal disease: systematic review and meta-analysis. J Clin Periodontol. 2016;43:492–502.

De Oliveira NF, Andia DC, Planello AC, Pasetto S, Marques MR, Nociti FH Jr, et al. TLR2 and TLR4 gene promoter methylation status during chronic periodontitis. J Clin Periodontol. 2011;38:975–83.

Duarte PM, da Rocha M, Sampaio E, et al. Serum levels of cytokines in subjects with generalized chronic and aggressive periodontitis before and after non-surgical periodontal therapy: a pilot study. J Periodontol. 2010;81:1056–63.

Ebersole JL, Schuster JL, Stevens J, Dawson D 3rd, Kryscio RJ, Lin Y, Thomas MV, Miller CS. Patterns of salivary analytes provide diagnostic capacity for distinguishing chronic adult periodontitis from health. J Clin Immunol. 2013;33:271–9.

Eke PI, Dye BA, Wei L, Thornton-Evans GO, Genco RJ, CDC Periodontal Disease Surveillance workgroup, James Beck, G. D. R. P. Prevalence of periodontitis in adults in the United States: 2009 and 2010. J Dent Res. 2012;91:914–20.

Finoti LS, Nepomuceno R, Pigossi SC, Corbi SCT, Secolin R, Scarel-Caminaga RM. Association between interleukin-8 levels and chronic periodontal disease. A PRISMA-compliant systematic review and meta-analysis. Medicine. 2017;96(22):e6932.

Franco C, Patricia HR, Sorsa T, et al. Matrix metalloproteinases as regulators of periodontal inflammation. Int J Mol Sci. 2017;18:E440.

Frodge BD, Ebersole JL, Kryscio RJ, Thomas MV, Miller CS. Bone remodelling biomarkers of periodontal disease in saliva. J Periodontol. 2008;79:1913–9.

Gemmell E, Yamazaki A, Seymour GJ. The role of T cells in periodontal disease: homeostasis and autoimmunity. Periodontol 2000. 2007;43:14–40.

Ghallab NA. Diagnostic potential and future directions of biomarkers in gingival crevicular fluid and saliva of periodontal diseases: review of the current evidence. Arch Oral Biol. 2018;87:115–24.

Ghallab N, Shaker O. Salivary-soluble CD44 levels in smokers and non-smokers with chronic periodontitis: a pilot study. J Periodontol. 2010;81:710–7.

Gheren LW, Cortelli JR, Rodrigues E, Holzhausen M, Saad WA. Periodontal therapy reduces arginase activity in saliva of patients with chronic periodontitis. Clin Oral Investig. 2008;12:67–72.

Giannobile WV. C-telopeptide pyridinoline cross-links. Sensitive indicators of periodontal tissue destruction. Ann N Y Acad Sci. 1999;878:404–12.

Giannobile WV, Beikler T, Kinney JS, Ramseier CA, Morelli T, Wong DT. Saliva as a diagnostic tool for periodontal disease. Current state and future directions. Periodontol. 2009;50:52–64.

Graves DT, Cochran D. The contribution of interleukin-1 and tumor necrosis factor to periodontal tissue destruction. J Periodontol. 2013;74:391–401.

Gul SS, Griffiths GS, Stafford GP, Al-Zubidi MI, Rawlinson A, Douglas CWI. Investigation of a novel predictive biomarker profile for the outcome of periodontal treatment. J Periodontol. 2017;88:1135–44.

Gümüş P, Nizam N, Lappin DF, Buduneli N. Saliva and serum levels of B-cell activating factors and tumor necrosis factor-a in patients with periodontitis. J Periodontol. 2014a;85:270–80.

Gümüş P, Nizam N, Nalbantsoy A, Özçaka Ö, Buduneli N. Saliva and serum levels of pentraxin-3 and interleukin-1β in generalised aggressive or chronic periodontitis. J Periodontol. 2014b;85:e40–6.

Gümüş P, Nizam N, Nalbantsoy A, Özçaka Ö, Buduneli N. Saliva, serum levels of interleukin-21, −33 and prostaglandin E2 in patients with generalised aggressive or chronic periodontitis. Oral Health Prev Dent. 2017;15:385–90.

Gupta M, Chaturvedi R, Jain A. Role of monocyte chemoattractant protein-1 (MCP-1) as an immune diagnostic biomarker in the pathogenesis of chronic periodontal disease. Cytokine. 2013;61:892–7.

Gürlek Ö, Gümüş P, Nile CJ, Lappin DF, Buduneli N. Biomarkers and bacteria around implants and natural teeth in the same individuals. J Periodontol. 2017;88:752–61.

Haffajee AD, Socransky SS, Goodson JM. Clinical parameters as predictors of destructive periodontal disease activity. J Clin Periodontol. 1983;10:257–65.

Hajishengallis G. Immunomicrobial pathogenesis of periodontitis: keystones, pathobionts, and host response. Trends Immunol. 2014;35:3–11.

Hajishengallis E, Hajishengallis G. Neutrophil homeostasis and periodontal health in children and adults. J Dent Res. 2014;93:231–7.

Heikkenen AM, Nwhator SO, Rathnayake N, Mantyla P, Vatanen P, Sorsa T. Pilot study on oral health status as assessed by an active matrix metalloproteinase-8 chairside mouthrinse test in adolescents. J Periodontol. 2016;87:36–40.

Heikkenen AM, Raivisto T, Kettunen K, Kovanen L, Haukka J, Esmaeili EP, et al. Pilot study on the genetic background of an active matrix metalloproteinase (aMMP-8) test in Finnish adolescents. J Periodontol. 2017;88:464–72.

Hernandez M, Vernal R, Sorsa T, Tervahartiala T, Mantyla P, Gamonal J. The role of immune-inflammatory response in the pathogenesis of chronic periodontitis and development of chair-side point-of-care diagnostics. In: Buduneli N, editor. Pathogenesis and treatment of periodontitis. London: InTech Publishing Co.; 2012. p. 33–54.

Iwakura Y, nakae S, Saijo S, Ishigame H. The roles of IL-17A in inflammatory immune responses and host defense against pathogens. Immunol Rev. 2008;226:57–79.

Kagiya T. MicroRNAs and osteolytic bone metastasis: the roles of microRNAs in tumor-induced osteoclast differentiation. J Clin Med. 2015;4:1741–52.

Kagiya T. MicroRNAs: potential biomarkers and therapeutic targets for alveolar bone loss in periodontal disease. Int J Mol Sci. 2016;17:1317.

Kaman WE, Galassi F, de Soet JJ, Bizzarro S, Loos BG, Veerman EC, et al. Highly specific protease-based approach for detection of *Porphyromonas gingivalis* in diagnosis of periodontitis. J Clin Microbiol. 2012;50:104–12.

Kassebaum NJ, Bernabé E, Dahiya M, Bhandari B, Murray CJ, Marcenes W. Global burden of severe periodontitis in 1990-2010: a systematic review and meta-regression. J Dent Res. 2014;93:1045–53.

Kathariya R, Jain H, Gujar D, Singh A, Ajwani H, Mandhyan D. Pentraxins as key disease markers for periodontal diagnosis. Dis Markers. 2013;34:143–51.

Kaufman E, Lamster IB. Analysis of saliva for periodontal diagnosis–a review. J Clin Periodontol. 2000;27:453–65.

Khan AI, Kerfoot SM, Heit B, et al. Role of CD44 and hyaluronan in neutrophil recruitment. J Immunol. 2004;173:7594–601.

Kinane DF. Regulators of tissue destruction and homeostasis as diagnostic aids in periodontology. Periodontol. 2009;24:215–25.

Kinane DF, Peterson M, Stathopoulou PG. Environmental and other modifying factors of the periodontal diseases. Periodontol. 2006;40:107–19.

Korn T, Bettelli E, Oukka M, Kuchroo VK. IL-17 and Th17 cells. Annu Rev Immunol. 2009;27:485–517.

Köseoğlu S, Sağlam M, Pekbağrıyanık T, Savran L, Sütcü R. Level of IL-35 in gingival crevicular fluid, saliva and plasma in periodontal disease and health. J Periodontol. 2015;19:1–12.

Lamster IB, Kaufman E, Grbic JT, Winston IJ, Singer RE. B-glucuronidase activity in saliva: relationship to clinical periodontal parameters. J Periodontol. 2003;74:353–9.

Leppilahti JM, Kallio MA, Tervahartiala T, Sorsa T, Mantyla P. Gingival crevicular fluid matrix metalloproteinase-8 levels predict treatment outcome among smokers with chronic periodontitis. J Periodontol. 2014a;85:250–60.

Leppilahti JM, Hernandez-Rios P, Gamonal JA, Tervahartiala T, Brignardello-Petersen R, Mantyla P, Sorsa T, Hernandez M. Matrix metalloproteinases and myeloperoxidase in gingival crevicular fluid provide site-specific diagnostic value for chronic periodontitis. J Clin Periodontol. 2014b;41:348–56.

Lester SR, Bain JL, Johnson RB, Serio FG. Gingival concentrations of interleukin-23 and -17 at healthy sites and at sites of clinical attachment loss. J Periodontol. 2007;78:1545–50.

Lindroth AM, Park YJ. Epigenetic biomarkers: A step forward for understanding periodontitis. J Periodontal Implant Sci. 2013;43:111–20.

Loesche WJ, Lopatin DE, Giordano J, et al. Comparsion of the benzoyl-DL-argininenaphtylamide (BANA) test, DNA probes, and immunological reagents for ability to detect anaerobic periodontal infections due to *Porphyromonas gingivalis, Treponema denticola,* and *Bacteroides forsythus*. J Clin Microbiol. 1992;30:427–33.

Loo WT, Jin L, Cheung MN, Wang M, Chow LW. Epigenetic change in E-cadherin and COX-2 to predict chronic periodontitis. J Transl Med. 2010;8:110.

Loos BG, Tjoa S. Host-derived diagnostic markers for periodontitis: do they exist in gingival crevice fluid? Periodontol. 2005;39:53–72.

Lorenzo-Poso AI, Perez-Sayans M, Bravo SB, Lopez-Jornet P, Garcia-Vence M, Alonso-Sampedro M, Carballo J. Protein-based salivary profiles as novel biomarkers for oral diseases. Dis Markers. 2018;2018:6141845.

Lu HK, Chen YL, Chang HC, Li CL, Kuo MY. Identification of the osteoprotegerin/receptor activator of nuclear factor-kappa B ligand system in gingival crevicular fluid and tissue of patients with chronic periodontitis. J Periodontal Res. 2006;41:354–60.

Mantyla P, Stenman M, Kinane DF, Tikanoja S, Luoto H, Salo T, Sorsa T. Gingival crevicular fluid collagenase-2 (matrix metalloproteinase-8) test stick for chair-side monitoring of periodontitis. J Periodontal Res. 2003;38:436–9.

Marcaccini AM, Meschiari CA, Sorgi CA, et al. Circulating interleukin-6 and high-sensitivity C-reactive protein decrease after periodontal therapy in otherwise healthy subjects. J Periodontol. 2009a;80:594–602.

Marcaccini AM, Novaes AB, Jr Meschiari CA, et al. Circulating matrix metalloproteinase-8 (MMP-8) and MMP-9 are increased in chronic periodontal disease and decrease after non-surgical periodontal therapy. Clin Chim Acta. 2009b;409:117–22.

Marcaccini AM, Meschiari CA, Zuardi LR, et al. Gingival crevicular fluid levels of MMP-8, MMP-9, TIMP-2 and MPO decrease after periodontal therapy. J Clin Periodontol. 2010;37:180–90.

Miller CS, Foley JD, Bailey AL, et al. Current development in salivary diagnostics. Biomark Med. 2010;4:171–89.

Mogi M, Otogoto J, Ota N, Togari A. Differential expression of RANKL and osteoprotegerin in gingival crevicular fluid of patients with periodontitis. J Dent Res. 2004;83:166–9.

Mombelli A. Critical issues in periodontal diagnosis. Periodontol. 2005;39:9–12.

Monteleone G, Pallone F, Macdonald TT. Interleukin-25: a two-edged sword in the control of immune-inflammatory responses. Cytokine Growth Factor Rev. 2010;21:471–5.

Nagase H. Activation mechanisms of matrix metalloproteinases. Biol Chem. 1997;378:151–60.

Nakajima T, Honda T, Domon H, et al. Periodontitis-associated up-regulation of systemic inflammatory mediator level may increase the risk of coronary heart disease. J Periodontal Res. 2010;45:116–22.

Nizam N, Gümüş P, Pitkanen J, Tervahartiala T, Sorsa T, Buduneli N. Serum and salivary matrix metalloproteinases, neutrophil elastase, myeloperoxidase in patients with chronic or aggressive periodontitis. Inflammation. 2014;37:1771–8.

Nussbaum G, Shapira L. How has neutrophil research improved our understanding of periodontal pathogenesis? J Clin Periodontol. 2011;38:49–59.

O'Brien-Simpson NM, Burgess K, Brammar GC, et al. Development and evaluation of a saliva-based chair-side diagnostic for the detection of *Porphyromonas gingivalis*. J Oral Microbiol. 2015;7:29129.

Offenbacher S, Beck JD, Moss K, et al. Results from the periodontitis and vascular events (PAVE) study: a pilot multicentered, randomized, controlled trial to study effects of periodontal therapy in a secondary prevention model of cardiovascular disease. J Periodontol. 2009;80:190–201.

Oliveira NF, Damm GR, Andia DC, Salmon C, Nociti FH Jr, Line SR, et al. DNA methylation status of the IL8 gene promoter in oral cells of smokers and non-smokers with chronic periodontitis. J Clin Periodontol. 2009;36:719–25.

Özçaka Ö, Nalbantsoy A, Köse T, Buduneli N. Plasma osteoprotegerin levels are decreased in smoker chronic periodontitis patients. Aust Dent J. 2010;55:405–10.

Özçaka Ö, Nalbantsoy A, Buduneli N. Interleukin-17 and interleukin-18 levels in saliva and plasma of patients with chronic periodontitis. J Periodontal Res. 2011;46:592–8.

Özmeriç N. Advances in periodontal disease markers. Clin Chim Acta. 2014;343:1–16.

Paredes-Sanchez E, Montiel-Company JM, Iranzo-Cortes JE, Almerich-Torres T, Bellot-Arcis C, Almerich-Silla JM. Meta-analysis of the use of 8-OHdG in saliva as a marker of periodontal disease. Dis Markers. 2018;2018:7916578.

Paster BJ, Boches SK, Galvin JL, et al. Bacterial diversity in human subgingival plaque. J Bacteriol. 2001;183:3770–83.

Pelletier M, Maggi L, Micheletti A. al. Evidence for a cross-talk between human neutrophils and Th17 cells. Blood. 2010;115:335–43.

Pradeep AR, TM S, Garima G, Raju A. Serum levels of oncostatin M (a gp 130 cytokine): an inflammatory biomarker in periodontal disease. Biomarkers. 2010;15:277–82.

Prakasam S, Srinivasan M. Evaluation of salivary biomarker profiles following non-surgical management of chronic periodontitis. Oral Dis. 2014;20:171–7.

Ramseier CA, Kinney JS, Herr AE, Braun T, Sugai JV, Shelburne CA, Rayburn LA, Tran HM, Singh AK, Giannobile WV. Identification of pathogen and host-response markers correlated with periodontal disease. J Periodontol. 2009;80:436–46.

Rathnayake N, Gieselmann D-R, Heikkinen AM, Tervahartiala T, Sorsa T. Salivary diagnostics-point-of-care diagnostics of MMP-8 in dentistry and medicine. Diagnostics. 2017;7:7.

Renvert S, Lindahl C, Roos-Jansaker AM, Lessem J. Short-term effects of an anti-inflammatory treatment on clinical parameters and serum levels of C-reactive protein and proinflammatory cytokines in subjects with periodontitis. J Periodontol. 2009;80:892–900.

Romero AM, Mastromatteo-Alberga P, Escalona I, Correnti M. MMP-3 and MMP-8 levels in patients with chronic periodontitis before and after non-surgical periodontal therapy. Investig Clin. 2013;54:138–48.

Ryder MI. Comparison of neutrophil functions in aggressive and chronic periodontitis. Periodontol 2000. 2010;53:124–37.

Sahingur SE, Cohen RE. Analysis of host responses and risk for disease progression. Periodontol 2000. 2004;34:57–83.

Sanchez GA, Miozza VA, Delgado A, Busch I. Salivary IL-1b and PGE2 as biomarkers of periodontal status before and after periodontal treatment. J Clin Periodontol. 2013;40:1112–7.

Shibuya M. Vascular endothelial growth factor and its receptor system: physiological functions in angiogenesis and pathological roles in various diseases. J Biochem. 2013;153:13–9.

Socransky SS, Haffajee AD. Dental biofilms: difficult therapeutic targets. Periodontol. 2002;28:12–55.

Suda T, Takahashi N, Udagawa N, Jimi E, Gillespie MT, Martin TJ. Modulation of osteoclast differentiation and function by the new members of the tumor necrosis factor receptor and ligand families. Endocr Rev. 1999;20:345–57.

Taba M Jr, Kinney J, Kim AS, Giannobile WV. Diagnostic biomarkers for oral and periodontal diseases. Dent Clin N Am. 2005;49:551.

Tobon-Arroyave SI, Jaramillo-Gonzales PE, Isaza-Guzman DM. Correlation between salivary IL-b levels and periodontal clinical status. Arch Oral Biol. 2008;53:346–52.

Tsuchida S, Satoh M, Takiwaki M, Nomura F. Current status of proteomic technologies for discovering and identifying gingival crevicular fluid biomarkers for periodontal disease. Int J Mol Sci. 2019;20:86.

Türer CC, Durmuş D, Ballı U, Güven B. Effect of non-surgical periodontal treatment on gingival crevicular fluid and serum endocan, vascular endothelial growth factor-a, and tumor necrosis factor-alpha levels. J Periodontol. 2017;88:493–501.

van der Veen MH, Volgenant CM, Keijser B, Ten Cate JB, Crielaard W. Dynamics of red fluorescent dental plaque during experimental gingivitis-a cohort study. J Dent. 2016;48:71–6.

Wara-aswapati N, Surarit R, Chayasadom A, Boch JA, Pitiphat W. RANKL upregulation associated with periodontitis and *Porphromonas gingivalis*. J Periodontol. 2007;78:1062–9.

Wen H, Schaller MA, Dou Y, Hogaboam CM, Kunkel SL. Dendritic cells at the interface of innate and acquired immunity: the role for epigenetic changes. J Leukoc Biol. 2008;83:439–46.

Yoshie H, Tai H, Kobayashi T, et al. Salivary enzyme levels after scaling and interleukin-1 genotypes in Japanese patients with chronic periodontitis. J Periodontol. 2007;78:498–503.

Zhang S, Crivello A, Offenbacher S, Moretti A, Paquette DW, Barros SP. Interferon-gamma promoter hypomethylation and increased expression in chronic periodontitis. J Clin Periodontol. 2010;37:953–61.

Zhang S, Barros SP, Moretti A, Yu N, Zhou J, Preisser JS, et al. Epigenetic regulation of TNFA expression in periodontal disease. J Periodontol. 2013;84:1606–16.

Zhang L, Li X, yan H, Huang L. Salivary matrix metalloproteinase (MMP)-8 as a biomarker for periodontitis. A PRISMA-compliant systematic review and meta-analysis. Medicine. 2018;97(3):e9642.

Zhuo L, Kanamori A, Kannagi R, et al. SHAP potentiates the CD44-mediated leukocyte adhesion to the hyaluronan substratum. J Biol Chem. 2006;281:20303–14.

6 Biological Samples for Biomarkers: Strengths and Weaknesses

Various biological samples have been used so far as candidate sources of biomarkers for diagnosis of periodontal diseases. Saliva is a commonly used biofluid sample that can be regarded as a source of information both at local and systemic levels. Gingival crevicular fluid (GCF) is the most specific biofluid that can be sampled for diagnosis and monitoring of the follow-up for periodontal diseases. Serum or plasma samples can give information about the diagnosis as well as aetiology related particularly with systemic factors. Biopsy of soft tissue in terms of gingiva can provide also valuable information and in some certain cases, biopsy of calcified tissue can be considered. Supragingival or subgingival plaque samples are also valuable for diagnostic purposes. Sampling of biological samples is usually technique-sensitive. All these biological samples have their own positive and negative aspects.

6.1 Saliva

Saliva is produced by the major and minor salivary glands, its secretion has critical physiological functions and it is a key component of the host defence against the microbial attacks from the dental biofilm. Information on the host immune response as well as pathogen microbiota can be provided. Saliva is becoming more and more popular as a diagnostic biofluid not only for oral diseases but also for systemic diseases such as diabetes mellitus. Nowadays, saliva is considered as the mirror of oral and systemic health (Kim et al. 2013). The main reasons behind its popularity can be outlined as follows: saliva is readily available, its collection does not require any specific instruments or skilled personnel, its collection is non-invasive making its sampling well received by most of the patients, usually it can be collected in sufficient volumes appropriate for quantitative analysis of multiple parameters, it is convenient for repetitive sampling for follow-up purposes, it has a very wide panel of content deriving from serum, gingival crevicular fluid, dental biofilm, and nutrients. It reflects a consensus of whole mouth inflammatory status (Lehner 1992; Buduneli and Kinane 2011; Jaedicke et al. 2016). Thus, salivary analysis has a great potential in large clinical trials, epidemiological studies, in self-management of disease even in circumstances where access to clinical facilities is scarce (Kaufman and Lamster 2000; Zhang et al. 2009; Kinney et al. 2011).

The major salivary glands are the parotid, submandibular, and sublingual glands. The minor salivary glands are minor sublingual, labial, buccal, glossopalatinal, palatinal, and lingual glands. Saliva has multiple functions such as food digestion, the perception of taste, and protection of oral tissues against chemical, physical, microbiological irritants. Healthy individuals normally secrete 600–1500 mL of saliva daily depending

N. Buduneli, *Biomarkers in Periodontal Health and Disease*,
https://doi.org/10.1007/978-3-030-37317-7_6

on the presence or absence of stimulation, where the average volume for a day is 1000 mL (Lindhe et al. 1997). Its secretion rate is the least during the sleep and the secretion rate can vary from 0.3–0.5 mL/min to 1–3 mL/min depending on the amount of stimulation. Most of the saliva (80–90% of daily salivary production) is secreted upon stimulation that is related with nutrition, taste and smell of foods, and the act of mastication. Approximately 90% of the saliva comes from the parotid and submandibular glands, 5% from the sublingual gland, and the other 5% from the minor salivary glands. Saliva has a relative density of 1.004–1.009. The pH of normal saliva is neutral that differs between 6.8 and 7.2. It is slightly acidic before secretion and becomes slightly alkaline after secretion due to loosing CO_2.

6.1.1 Collection of Saliva Samples

Saliva can be sampled as the whole saliva or as specific samples directly from the specific salivary glands. Whole saliva sampling: Whole saliva is usually obtained by simply having the patient expectorate into sterile tubes. Patients should refrain from eating, drinking, and plaque control measures at least 1 h before collection of whole saliva. It is also recommended that patients rinse their mouth with deionised water just before whole saliva collection. It can be stimulated or unstimulated. Chewing gum, hard plastic, or paraffin can be used for mechanical stimulation of saliva secretion. Alternatively, putting a few drops of citric acid on the tongue dorsum provides taste stimuli for the rapid secretion. There are also pharmacologic and electric stimulants. Collecting whole saliva is easy and fast, but it has a complex nature and contains extraoral substances such as food debris as well. Unstimulated saliva samples can be obtained by passive drooling of the resting saliva from the floor of the mouth into a graduated tube or preweighed vial so that flow rate per unit time can be measured and this draining method is regarded as the gold standard. Apart from spitting and draining whole saliva samples can be obtained by suction and using the swab method (Navazesh 1993). Various devices are available for collection of unstimulated whole saliva that are Salivette® (Sarstedt, Nümbrecht, Germany), Quantisal® (Immunalysis, Pomona, CA, USA), Orapette® (Trinity Biotech, Dublin, Ireland), SCS® (Greiner Bio-One, Kremsmünster, Austria) (Khurshid et al. 2016). Unstimulated saliva is preferred, as it contains higher concentrations of biomarkers and can provide more information.

Parotid saliva: In some cases, specific saliva samples can be necessary rather than the whole saliva sample. This can be obtained directly from the Stensen canal of the parotid gland using special instruments. It can also be stimulated or unstimulated.

Saliva secretion is controlled by the saliva centre in the medulla. The majority of the control is parasympathetic but there is also sympathetic control. The proprioceptors in the periodontal ligament and masticatory muscles act in the control of saliva secretion.

Xerostomia or dry mouth defines the insufficient amounts of saliva. This can occur due to the obturation of salivary gland canals, some drug effects, radiotherapy, and psychological disorders. Dry mouth can increase accumulation of food debris, materia alba, and microbial dental plaque in the dentate individuals eventually increasing the risk of carious as well as inflammatory periodontal diseases (Genco et al. 1990). On the other hand, edentulous individuals with dry mouth have difficulty in wearing the dentures. The oral mucosa becomes dry and sticky and bleeds more easily. The tongue surface looks reddish, flattened, thin, and more vulnerable to mechanical irritations. The taste perception is usually decreased. Mouth breathing also dries the intraoral surfaces and increases the risk of gingivitis.

Various drugs used frequently in the elderly people such as barbiturates, antihistaminic drugs, atropine-like agents, psychoactive agents, and antihypertensive drugs may also cause dry mouth, thereby leading to taste deficiency, cervical carious lesions, and root decays.

6.1.2 Content of Saliva

Saliva content comes from various sources (Fig. 6.1). Saliva is composed of 99% water, 0.3% proteins, and 0.2% organic and inorganic components. Among these organic substances, there are antibodies, lipids, ammonia, uric acid, glucose, glycoproteins, enzymes, urea, etc. The concentrations of glucose, amino acids, and lipids are very low. The inorganic components are electrolytes and various elements such as K^+, Ca^{+2}, Na^+, Cl^-, and HCO_3^-. Gases like CO_2, O_2, NO_2 are present in the form of melted in water. Moreover, there are hundreds of microorganisms.

Saliva has a significant antioxidant capacity because of the enzymes (i.e., salivary peroxidase, superoxide dismutase, catalase, glutathione peroxidase, myeloperoxidase), uric acid, ascorbic acid, and also albumin (Battino et al. 2002; Zukowski et al. 2018) and acts as the first line of defence against oxidative stress, reactive oxygen species, and free radicals. Protein content of saliva can be divided into eight groups as follows: buffering proteins (carbonic anhydrases, histatins); digestive proteins (amylases, mucins, lipases); mineralisation proteins (cystatins, histatins, proline-rich proteins, statherins); proteins related with viscoelasticity and lubrication (mucins and statherins); tissue coating proteins (amylase, cystatins, mucins, proline-rich proteins, statherins); anti-fungal proteins (lactoferrin, peroxidases, immunoglobulins, mucins, histatins); anti-viral proteins (mucins, lactoferrin, cystatins, immunoglobulins, peroxidases); and antibacterial proteins (amylases, cystatins, histatins, mucins, peroxidases, lactoferrin, lysozyme, agglutinin) (Van Nieuw Amerongen et al. 2004).

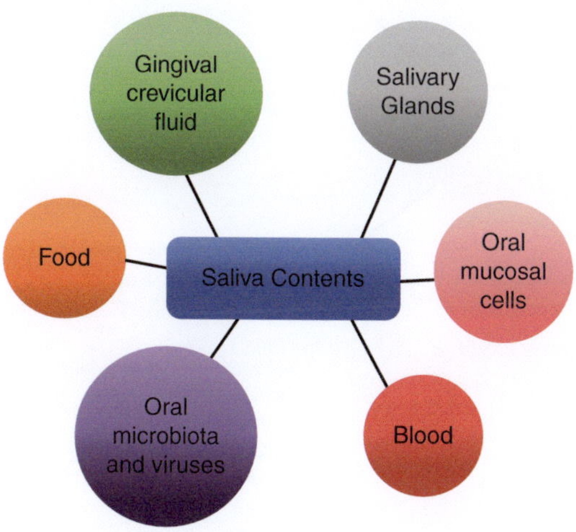

Fig. 6.1 Sources for saliva contents

Saliva has a significant concentration of secretory immunoglobulin A (sIgA), which tends to increase by the increasing age (Tenovuo 1998). This antibody is effective against the viruses, bacterial antigens, and even some antigens coming from nutrients. Lysozyme is another antibacterial factor coming from the parotid and submaxillary glands. Sialoperoxidase is also an antibacterial agent.

Other proteins in saliva are acid and alkaline phosphatases, nonspecific esterase, ribonucleic acid, and callikrein. Moreover, there is also cellular content comprising mainly the desquamated epithelial cells and leukocytes. Approximately 98–99% of leukocytes are polymorphonuclear leukocytes, 1% is lymphocytes. There are also some monocytes and eosinophils. More than 2000 different proteins and enzymes have been identified in saliva samples so far (Priyanka et al. 2012).

6.1.3 Functions of Saliva

Saliva lubricates the oral surfaces so that speech and swallowing can be possible. Its constant flow is an important protective function. The glycoproteins and mucoids provide a protective layer on the oral mucosa against the proteolytic and hydrolytic enzymes, potential carcinogens (tobacco and chemical agents), and the dryness due to mouth breathing.

Saliva creates a surface tension on the oral surfaces and its antimicrobial content mainly the sIgA decreases the adhesion of various microorganisms to the tooth and mucosa surfaces. Thus, microorganisms can be swallowed and removed much easily from the oral cavity.

Saliva production can show individual variation and the content as well as the volume may be affected by factors such as circadian rhythm, diet, and oral hygiene habits.

Certain factors can affect the laboratory analysis findings and should be taken into account when evaluating the data reported. These are centrifugation speed, addition of protease inhibitors, and storage temperature as well as storage time, if required, transfer conditions. Ideally collected samples should be placed on ice and put in the freezer as soon as possible, not later than 1 h after collection and stored at the coldest possible conditions.

Key factors about saliva as a source for biomarkers:

- readily accessible
- non-invasive
- can be unstimulated or stimulated
- can be whole or specific
- mirror of the body
- has circadian rhythm
- >2000 proteins identified

6.2 Gingival Crevicular Fluid

Gingival crevicular fluid (GCF) is a physiological fluid that is defined as a serum transudate or an inflammatory exudate of the periodontal tissues in health and disease, respectively (Fig. 6.2). Transudate is the result of increased pressure in the veins and capillaries that forces interstitial fluid through the vessel walls into the crevice (Pashley 1976; Del Fabbro et al. 2001). It is a transudate because it is present even in pristine health state. Some researchers consider it as an exudate as it contains immune cells and its flow rate increases with gingival inflammation. Exudate is the result of increased permeability of the vessels underlying the junctional epithelium, allowing plasma to leak into the crevice (Griffiths 2003).

GCF is accepted as the most promising biofluid as a source of biochemical disease indicators as well as microbiological aetiological factors (Bostanci and Belibasakis 2018). However, in a specific cohort study comprising 100 patients over a 12-month period, GCF alone provided low sensitivity (23%) and high specificity (95%) values (Kinney et al. 2014). When combined with plaque pathogens, GCF biomarkers demonstrated the highest positive and negative predictive values, of 73% and 70%, respectively.

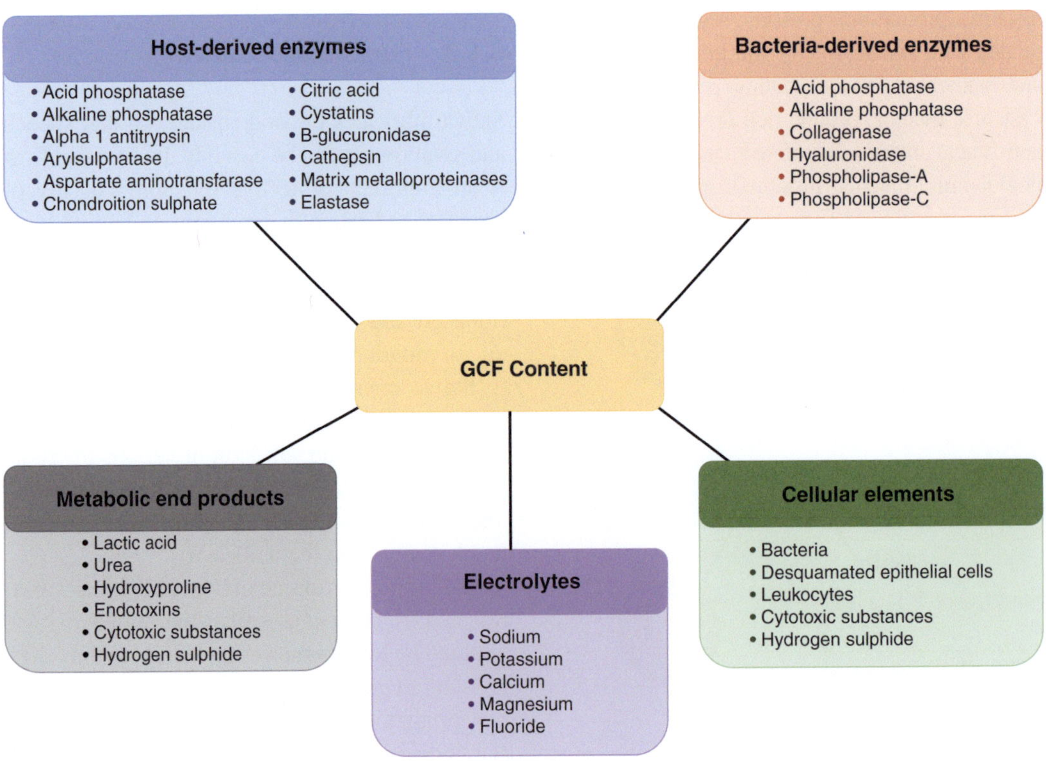

Fig. 6.2 GCF content

GCF originates from the blood vessels in the gingival connective tissue, subjacent to the sulcus/pocket epithelium (Griffiths 2003). Functions of GCF are as follows:

- cleaning materials from the sulcus by its constant flow,
- improving the adhesion of epithelium to tooth surface by the help of the plasma proteins it carries,
- acting in the defence of periodontal tissues by the antibodies and other antimicrobial factors in its content.

It has been discovered more than a century ago. It can be regarded as the most specific biofluid sample as it is obtained directly from the periodontal disease lesion. Investigations on host immune response as well as on microbiological aetiological factors can be performed in GCF samples.

GCF as a source for biomarkers:

- more than 400 proteins identified (Barros et al. 2016)
- more than 90 components (Loos and Tjoa 2005)
- more than 65 candidate biomarkers (Buduneli and Kinane 2011)

The content of GCF is very complex as the ingredients are coming from the serum, host tissues, and also from subgingival biofilm. GCF samples comprise leukocytes, desquamating epithelial cells, proteins, enzymes, tissue breakdown products, inflammatory mediators, and cytokines produced by the resident cells of blood cells (Armitage 2004). Loos and Tjoa (2005) reported that at least 90 different components have been investigated so far in three large categories:

1. Host-derived enzymes and their inhibitors.
2. Tissue breakdown products.
3. Inflammatory mediators and host modifiers.

The main disadvantage is the small quantity of the GCF sample particularly from the clinically healthy sites. The specific equipment and tools required for GCF sampling is considered as another

Table 6.1 Relationship between the GCF flow rate and gingival inflammation

Clinical periodontal diagnosis	GCF flow (μL/h)	Resting volume (μL/h)
Clinically healthy	3	0.05
Moderate pocketing	20	0.4
Deep pocketing	44	1.5

disadvantage. However, it is appropriate for repeated sampling for follow-up purposes and it is considered to offer a great potential to reflect the ongoing response of the periodontal cells towards the inflammatory agents (Barros et al. 2016).

In slightly inflamed sites, the amount of GCF sample was reported to be approximately 0.1 mg in 3 min of collection (Cimasoni 1983). A later study reported mean GCF sample volume ranging between 0.43 and 1.56 ml obtained from the interproximal aspects of molar teeth (Challacombe et al. 2007). Inflammation increases the flow of GCF. Smoking may cause a transient but remarkable increase in the GCF flow. The increase in sex steroid hormone levels during special periods like puberty, ovulation, and pregnancy causes an increase in GCF flow rate. GCF production also increases with mechanical stimulation and during the healing period after periodontal surgery. The flow rate or the sample volume itself may be considered as an indicator of gingival inflammation as outlined in Table 6.1.

Is there a circadian rhythm effect on GCF volume and/or content?

No support that GCF volume displays distinct daytime variations; rather demonstrate relatively stable GCF volumes between 08:00 and 18:00 (Günday et al. 2014).

6.2.1 Methods of Collection

6.2.1.1 Absorbent Paper Strips

1. Extracrevicular technique
2. Intracrevicular technique
   - orifice technique (just at the entrance of crevice/pocket),
   - deep intracrevicular technique (base of the pocket/until minimum resistance felt),
   - modified intracrevicular technique (exactly 1 mm into the pocket).

Using absorbent paper strips is the most common method of GCF collection. This technique is mostly preferred because it is easy, quick, and non-traumatic. It can be used for either extracrevicular or intracrevicular sampling. When the extracrevicular technique is used, the strip is placed on the tooth surface but not under the gingival margin (Fig. 6.3). The strip can be held in place for up to 2 min, but the most common duration is 30 s.

The intracrevicular technique has deep and superficial variations (Fig. 6.4). The sampling site is dried and isolated with cotton rolls and then in the deep intracrevicular technique, the absorbent filter paper is placed into the sulcus/pocket to a depth where a minimum resistance is felt by the strip from the base of the sulcus/pocket. On the other hand, by the superficial technique, the strip is placed approximately 1 mm below the gingival margin. The intracrevicular technique can provide a higher volume, whereas the extracrevicular technique provides a smaller volume.

There is a risk of contamination from blood or saliva; therefore, the proper isolation of the sampling site is of utmost importance. When there are visible signs of blood contamination, the strip is usually discarded, but lack of visible signs does not guarantee the lack of blood contamination. In case of severe gingival inflammation, it may not be possible to collect GCF sample due to severe bleeding even with minimal stimulation. In sites, where there is blood contamination, there should be an interval of at least 5 min between the repetitive samplings.

6.2.1.2 Gingival Washing Method

In this technique, the gingival crevice is perfused with a fixed volume of an isotonic solution, such as Hanks' balanced salt solution. The device used

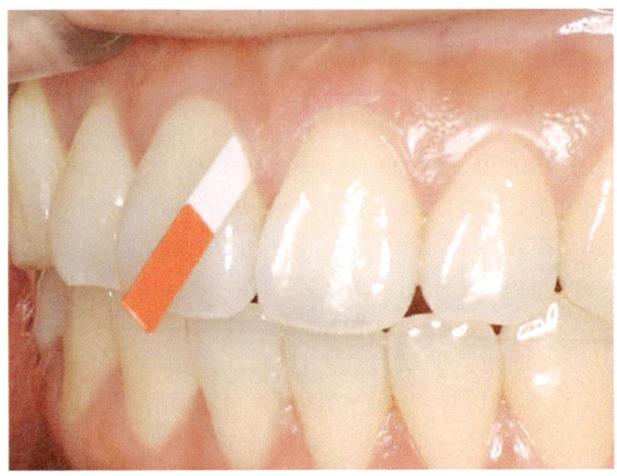

Fig. 6.4 The intracrevicular technique for GCF sampling

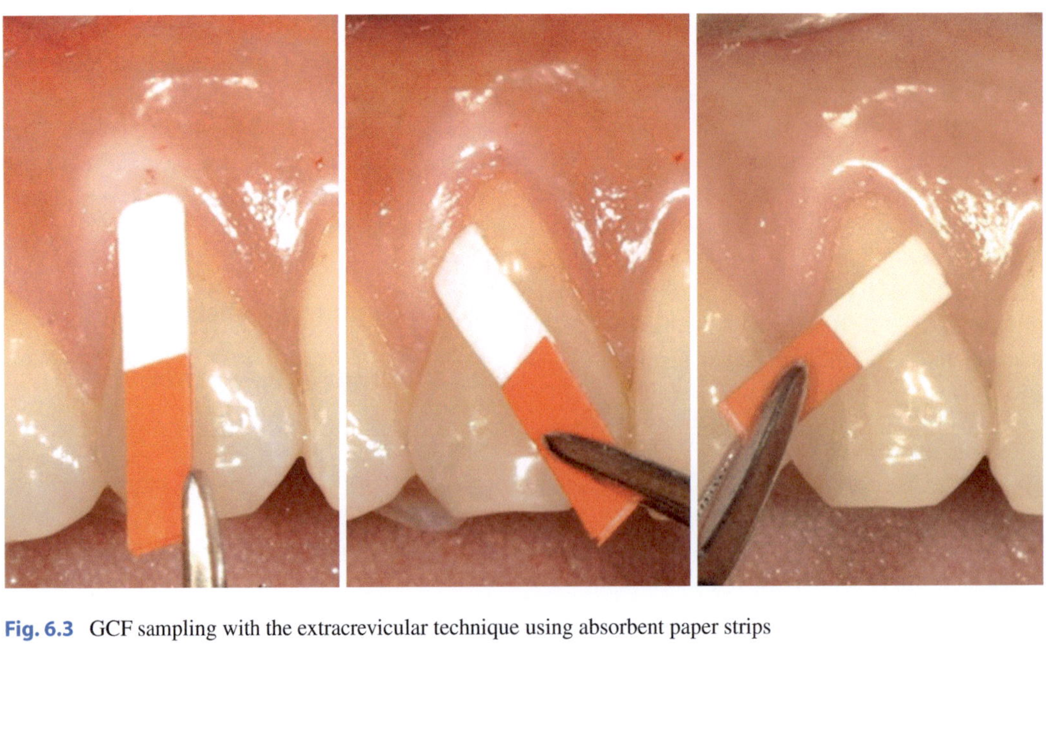

Fig. 6.3 GCF sampling with the extracrevicular technique using absorbent paper strips

to perform this method consists of two injection needles placed one inside the other (Salonen and Paunio 1991). This technique provides much higher sample volumes, but the fluid collected represents a dilution of GCF containing both cells and soluble plasma proteins. The washing technique is preferred particularly when the aim of sampling is focused more on cellular sources. However, it may not be possible to recollect the complete amount of the fluid; thus, the GCF sample volume and composition cannot be determined accurately as the precise dilution factor is not known.

6.2.1.3 Capillary Tubing or Micropipettes

In this technique, first the sampling site is isolated and dried, and then the capillary tubes of known internal diameter are inserted into the entrance of the gingival crevice. GCF migrates into the tube by capillary action. As the internal diameter of the capillary tube is known, the volume of the sample can be calculated by measuring the distance, which the GCF has migrated. This technique provides undiluted samples; however, the collection time may exceed 30 min. Moreover, recovering the complete sample from the tube may be difficult. An air jet or centrifugation of the tube are the most frequently used methods to recover the GCF sample from the tube.

6.2.2 Reporting GCF Sample Volume and Biomarker Data

The first step in the analysis is measuring the volume of the sample. Then the sample needs to be recovered/eluted if collected by absorbent paper strips. The GCF sample volume absorbed by filter paper strips can be quantified by electronic impedance using a special instrument (Periotron® ProFlow, Inc., Amityville, NY), which has to be calibrated regularly (Fig. 6.5). It has been reported that this instrument provides an accuracy of volume measurement within approximately 0.1–1.2 μL (Griffiths 2003). Volume measurement of the GCF sample is relevant as it usually increases with increasing gingival inflammation; thus, it is itself an indicator of inflammation.

The volume of the GCF sample is determined in terms of units and then transferred to microlitres by a standard curve. The recorded units give an idea about the clinical diagnosis (Table 6.2). Moreover, the biochemical data is reported either in terms of total amounts, that is, the quantity of the biochemical marker assayed per sampling time (e.g., pg per 30-s sample), or concentrations, that is, the quantity assayed per unit volume of GCF (e.g., pg/μL). Some researchers prefer reporting the data as concentrations. However, concentration data is severely affected by the sample volume and the less the sample volume, the higher the concentration of the biomarker.

Table 6.2 Relationship between the Periotron readings and gingival inflammation

Periotron reading (units)	Severity of gingival inflammation	Gingival index
0–20	Healthy	0
21–40	Mild	1
41–80	Moderate	2
81–200	Severe	3

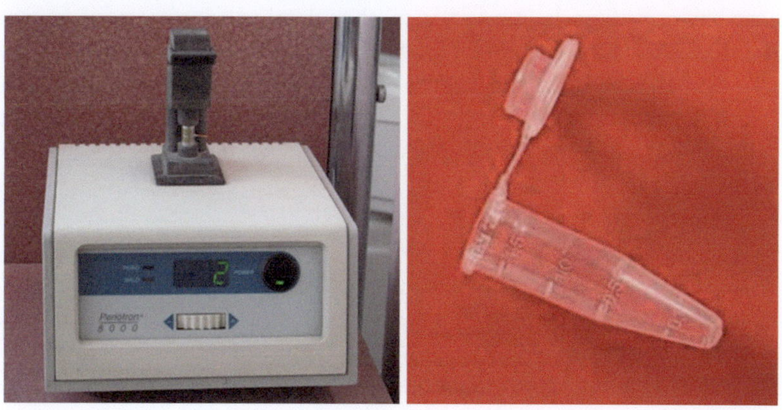

Fig. 6.5 Periotron 8000 and the dry Eppendorf tube that is usually used for GCF sample storage

This fact may lead to misinterpretations of the findings particularly in healthy control samples or when comparing data before and after periodontal treatment. Therefore, basing on total amounts rather than concentrations but reporting sample volumes may be more reliable. It is also common to report both total amounts and concentrations to allow readers evaluate the data in both ways.

It is also imperative in studies investigating GCF samples to fully explain the methodology of sample collection, storage conditions, elution, and laboratory analysis as all these steps have the potential to affect the findings. The recommended time of collection is before doing the periodontal probing, because probing may cause bleeding and contaminated GCF samples are to be discarded. It may be useful to know how many samples are contaminated and discarded and how many times sampling had to be repeated as well as the interval between the repeated samplings.

The volume of GCF sample should be preferentially measured and reported among the findings of the study.

GCF samples can be analysed individually or samples from different sites may be pooled in order to increase the sample volume. This issue should be clarified in the methods section of the study.

Placing the GCF sample in dry tubes or in buffer may also affect the results and therefore, it has to be stated.

The timing of elution is another factor and elution may be performed immediately after collection and before freezing or after freezing/thawing and before laboratory analysis. The protocol of eluting the GCF may also vary (shaking, vortexing, centrifuging, etc.). If samples are eluted by centrifuge, both g and r.p.m. should be reported. The limits of detection for the particular assay/kit should be given in the manuscript (Wassall and Preshaw 2016).

Important issues in GCF sample analysis:

- timing of sampling?
- is sample volume recorded?
- are samples assayed individually or pooled?
- storage; dry or in buffer?
- storage conditions?
- timing of elution? protocol for elution?
- lower and upper limits of detection?
- data handling and reporting?
- samples discarded due to contamination?

Table 6.3 Comparison of saliva and GCF as a biofluid for periodontal diagnostics

Fluid/parameters	Saliva	GCF
Collection difficulty	Easy	Easy/medium difficulty
Collected volume	High	Very low
Invasiveness	Non-invasive	Non-invasive/minimal
Collection speed	Fast	Fast
Contamination	Not applicable	Important (saliva, blood, plaque)
Relevancy	Less specific	Highly specific
Predictability of detection	High	Low
Site-specificity	–	+++
Sensitivity	+++	–
Healthy controls	Different individuals	The same individuals
Circadian rhythm	Yes	?

Saliva and GCF have different positive and negative aspects when compared as biofluids for potential biomarkers for periodontal diseases (Table 6.3).

6.3 Serum or Plasma

Peripheral blood samples can be obtained usually from the antecubital vein by a venipuncture and then depending on the aim of sampling, serum or plasma samples can be prepared. Circulating blood sample can be obtained at the required amount and can provide information on the systemic health state of the patient. Immune response against the periodontopathogens can be evaluated in blood samples by evaluating the levels of specific immunoglobulins. The main disadvantage is that it is invasive and may not be well received by all patients.

6.4 Gingival Tissue Biopsy

Gingival tissue biopsy can also provide valuable information on the present health state. Gingival tissue samples are usually obtained under local anaesthesia during periodontal surgical interventions, tooth extractions, or crown lengthening surgeries. However, it may not be possible to obtain tissue samples in all patients or from all sites. Furthermore, the amount of the sample may not be sufficient in all cases and it is not appropriate for repeated sampling from the same site.

6.5 Calcified Tissue Biopsy

Sample of calcified tissue may provide information for diagnosis of some particular diseases. It is also valuable for follow-up evaluations after regenerative periodontal surgery. However, it is invasive, can only be sampled during surgical intervention or re-entry, and may not be possible to do so in all patients or sites.

6.6 Plaque

Sampling of plaque is easy and can be repeated any time, as it is not invasive. Both supragingival and subgingival plaque samples can be obtained and provide complementary information. However, microbiological testing is not necessary for diagnosing gingivitis or periodontitis and just to confirm what a periodontal probe can easily reveal. Microbiological analysis is more appropriate to monitor patients after periodontal treatment. Periodontitis has a rather high recurrence rate particularly in those patients with insufficient home care. Repopulation of pathogenic bacteria is a basic step in recurrence and therefore, early detection of recolonisation may help to define patients and/or sites with a high risk of recurrence.

A practical and economic approach to sample major pathogens from the subgingival area is to pool samples from the deepest bleeding pockets in each quadrant (Mombelli et al. 1991). Site-specific sampling on the other hand is of less importance as a precursor for systemic antibiotic therapy but may provide additional diagnostic information.

Major goals of microbiological testing can be outlined as follows:

- to discriminate microorganisms acting in periodontal disease pathogenesis,
- to define susceptible individuals for antibiotic therapy and to select the most appropriate antibiotics,
- to screen vertical and horizontal transmission of periodontal pathogens among family members,
- to help to determine the endpoint of active periodontal treatment and to establish recall intervals for maintenance program (van Winkelhoff et al. 2000).

6.7 Conclusion

There are a variety of biologic samples that can be collected for diagnostic purposes in the field of periodontology. The particular biologic sample as well as the particular method of sampling should be chosen according to the specific purpose of sampling. Each biological sample has its own strong and weak aspects in terms of providing diagnostic information about periodontal diseases. The information that can be obtained is also related with the sampling and laboratory investigation techniques. The storage conditions are also important for the outcomes of biofluids sample analysis. Generally, the colder the better. Storing in liquid nitrogen (−196 °C) is the best option also because it displaces dissolved oxygen in the fluid phase. By this, oxidation of the biological sample and reaction with molecular H_2O can be prevented. Hence biological samples can be stored stable, undegraded, unoxidised, and unmodified by enzymes for long periods.

References

Armitage GC. Analysis of gingival crevice fluid and risk of progression of periodontitis. Periodontol. 2004;34:109–19.

Barros SP, Williams R, Offenbacher S, Morelli T. Gingival crevicular fluid as a source of biomarkers for periodontitis. Periodontol. 2016;70:53–64.

Battino M, Ferreiro MS, Gallardo I, Newman HN, Bullon P. The antioxidant capacity of saliva. J Clin Periodontol. 2002;29:189–94.

Bostanci N, Belibasakis GN. Gingival crevicular fluid and its immune mediators in the proteomic era. Periodontol. 2018;76:68–84.

Buduneli N, Kinane DF. Host-derived diagnostic markers related to soft tissue destruction and bone degradation in periodontitis. J Clin Periodontol. 2011;38(Suppl. 11):85–105.

Challacombe SJ, Russell MW, Hawkes J. Passage of intact IgG from plasma to the diagnosis of oral and systemic diseases. Ann N Y Acad Sci. 2007;1098:216–29.

Cimasoni G. Crevicular fluid updated. Monogr Oral Sci. 1983;12:1–152.

Del Fabbro M, Francetti L, Bulfamante G, Cribiu M, Mirerocchi G, Weinstein RL. Fluid dynamics of gingival tissues in transition from physiological condition to inflammation. J Periodontol. 2001;72:65–73.

Genco RJ, Goldman HM, Cohen DW. Contemporary periodontics. St. Louis: The Mosby Company; 1990. p. 117–21.

Griffiths GS. Formation, collection and significance of gingival crevicular fluid. Periodontol. 2003;31:32–42.

Günday S, Topcu AO, Ercan E, Yamalık N. Analysis of daytime variations in gingival crevicular fluid: a circadian periodicity? J Periodontol. 2014;85:e47–56.

Jaedicke KM, Preshaw PM, Taylor JJ. Salivary cytokines as biomarkers for periodontal diseases. Periodontol. 2016;70:164–83.

Kaufman E, Lamster IB. Analysis of saliva for periodontal diagnosis. A review. J Clin Periodontol. 2000;27:453–65.

Khurshid Z, Zohaib S, Najeeb S, Zafar M, Slowey P, Almas K. Human saliva collection devices for proteomics: an update. Int J Mol Sci. 2016;17:846.

Kim JJ, Kim CJ, Camargo PM. Salivary biomarkers in the diagnosis of periodontal diseases. J Calif Dent Assoc. 2013;41:119–24.

Kinney JS, Morelli T, Braun T, et al. Saliva/pathogen biomarker signatures and periodontal disease progression. J Dent Res. 2011;90:752–8.

Kinney JS, Morelli T, Oh M, Braun TM, Ramseier CA, Sugai JV, Giannobile WV. Crevicular fluid biomarkers and periodontal disease progression. J Clin Periodontol. 2014;41:113–20.

Lehner T. Immunology of oral diseases. 3rd ed. Oxford: Blackwell Scientific Publications; 1992. p. 9–17.

Lindhe J, Karring T, Lang NP. Clinical periodontology and implant dentistry. 3rd ed. Copenhagen: Munksgaard; 1997.

Loos BG, Tjoa S. Host-derived diagnostic markers for periodontitis: do they exist in gingival crevice fluid? Periodontol. 2005;39:53–72.

Mombelli A, McNabb H, Lang NP. Black-pigmenting gram-negative bacteria in periodontal disease. II. Screening strategies for detection of P gingivalis. J Periodontal Res. 1991;26:308–13.

Navazesh M. Methods for collecting saliva. Ann N Y Acad Sci. 1993;694:72–7.

Pashley DH. A mechanistic analysis of gingival fluid production. J Periodontal Res. 1976;11:121–34.

Priyanka N, Kalra N, Shanbhag N, Kumar K, Seema Brijet B, et al. Recent approaches in saliva as a credible periodontal diagnostic and prognostic marker. AOSR. 2012;2:40–6.

Salonen JI, Paunio KU. An intracrevicular washing method for collection of crevicular contents. Scand J Dent Res. 1991;99:406–12.

Tenovuo J. Antimicrobial function of human saliva—how important is it for oral health? Acta Odontol Scand. 1998;56:250–6.

Van Nieuw Amerongen A, Bolscher JGM, Veerman ECI. Salivary proteins: protective and diagnostic value in cariology? Caries Res. 2004;38:247–53.

van Winkelhoff AJ, Goene RJ, Benschop C, Folmer T. Early colonisation of dental implants by putative periodontal pathogens in partially edentulous patients. Clin Oral Implants Res. 2000;11:511–20.

Wassall RR, Preshaw PM. Clinical and technical considerations in the analysis of gingival crevicular fluid. Periodontol. 2016;70:65–79.

Zhang I, Henson BS, Camargo PM, Wong DT. The clinical value of salivary biomarkers for periodontal diseases. Periodontol. 2009;51:25–37.

Zukowski P, Maciejczyk M, Waszkiel D. Sources of free radicals and oxidative stress in the oral cavity. Arch Oral Biol. 2018;92:8–17.

Technologies for Biomarkers in Periodontics

7

7.1 Biochemical Analyses

There are different methods that have been used for detecting biomarkers for periodontal diseases. There are several sensitive analytical techniques that allow detection and quantification of a large number of biomarkers in saliva samples such as mass spectrometry (MS), reverse transcription-polymerase chain reaction (RT-PCR), micro-arrays, nano-scale sensors, magnetic resonance spectroscopy (MRS), western blot, immunoassay techniques, and enzymatic assays. The most prominent approaches are genomics, transcriptomics, proteomics, metabolomics, and metagenomics. However, it has to be remembered that the levels of transcripts, proteins, and metabolites may reflect not only the genetic programming, but also the consequences of the host response to the extrinsic factors together with factors related with the disease course.

Enzyme-linked immunosorbent assay (ELISA), bioassay, radioimmunoassay, radioimmunofluorescence, enzyme immunoassay (EIA), and spectrophotometer (SPM) are those used most frequently. Moreover, quantitative time-resolved immunofluorometric assay (IFMA), electrochemiluminescent technique, flow cytometry, western immunoblot assay, immunoturbidimetric analysis, checkerboard immunoblotting are also utilised while searching for biomarkers for periodontal diseases. ELISA is used very frequently as it is sensitive, cost-effective, and it has high throughput and high reproducibility (Jaedicke et al. 2016). ELISA is much more sensitive to detect pro-inflammatory and anti-inflammatory cytokines compared to MS (Fig. 7.1). Very small volumes of samples can be assayed by ELISA and it gives objective and numerical data. One parameter can usually be assayed by ELISA at a time in one GCF sample. ELISA technology has been improved and two basic multiple assays have been developed for simultaneous quantification of multiple parameters including planar array assays and microbead assays. By development of these multiplex assays based on a combination of antibody-coated beads mixed in a common solution, it became possible to quantify up to 500 different parameters in very small amount of biofluids as small as 50 μl and within a single experimental run (Wang et al. 2002). Following incubation with the sample, labelled detection antibodies are added into the system to bind onto the analyte captured onto the corresponding bead and are then passed through a flow-through detection and quantification system. Alternatively, cytokine antibody arrays use capture antibodies spotted onto nitrocellulose membranes instead of beads. These systems provide great advantages for biomarker search for periodontal diseases; however, they have high costs limiting their use in large clinical or observational studies (Wassall and Preshaw 2016).

N. Buduneli, *Biomarkers in Periodontal Health and Disease*,
https://doi.org/10.1007/978-3-030-37317-7_7

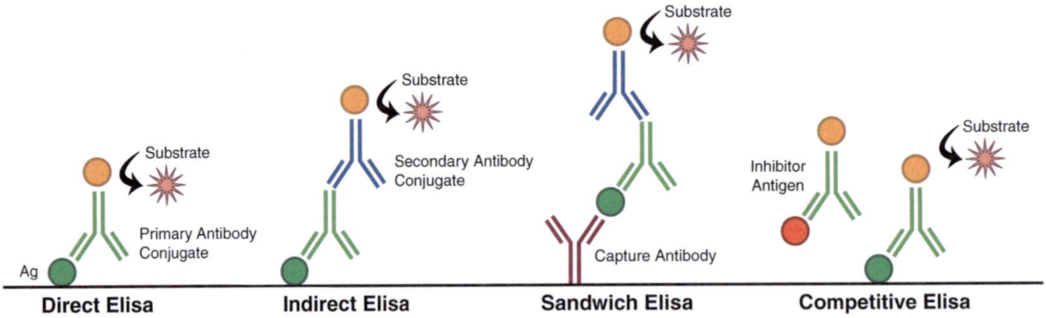

Fig. 7.1 Basic principle of ELISA

Moreover, multiplex immunoassays may provide only a small peek into the complex network of molecules that are present in the biofluids. Current attempts for improving mass spectrometry instrumentation together with the publicly available databases of every protein encoded and expressed by every human gene will allow for a more accurate assessment of the global protein content of biofluids such as GCF (Bostanci et al. 2010).

There are advantages and disadvantages of each technique and the technique to be used can be chosen by considering the following factors:

- accuracy and efficiency in biomarker detection and quantification,
- feasibility of the test,
- cost effectiveness,
- time required for the test,
- the particular purpose of the study.

Human saliva is a rich reservoir of proteins and peptides sharing approximately 51% of that of plasma (Lorenzo-Poso et al. 2018). Saliva has exosomes that are vesicles involved in intercellular traffic and highly stabile. Exosomes have genetic material (i.e., miRNAs) and also proteins and they play prominent roles in immune system modulation and inflammation (Spielmann and Wong 2011; Ogawa et al. 2011). Currently, there are five major branches of salivary analysis: proteomics, transcriptomics, microRNA (miRNA), metabolomics, and microbiomics (Kaczor-Urbanowicz et al. 2016).

7.1.1 Point-of-Care Diagnostics

Diagnostic targets using point-of-care (POC) technologies focus on small molecules such as nucleic acids, proteins, and metabolites. POC diagnostics is the medical testing that is performed right at the clinic or at the patient's home rather than in a laboratory. Optimally, they are chair-side tests or dip-stick tests. If patients can do such testing at home to diagnose periodontitis, then they can visit their dentist to seek treatment and accelerate treatment, thereby possibly decreasing the risk of progression of periodontitis and related tooth loss. Studies have been performed in GCF and saliva samples in an attempt to find explicit markers of periodontitis (Christodoulides et al. 2007; Miller et al. 2010; Giannobile 2012).

The advantages of POC tests are eliminating to draw blood and reducing the additional costs related with storage, shipment, and handling of samples in a specific laboratory. Having the assay result very rapidly is one of the most important advantages. Moreover, less training and fewer resources are required enabling screening of large populations in a short time. In this way, identification of risk groups can be done more effectively possibly increasing the access to treatment.

The disadvantages of POC tests are the need for validation for the specific biofluid sample and specific disease and their high cost. Clinicians look for diagnostic tests that will make a difference in their clinical routine and if this is not the case, then the diagnostic methods are not well accepted by most of the clinicians. Currently available chair-side tests brought information from bench to the chair but could not make an effect on the clinical practice so far (Sexton et al. 2011; Sackman et al. 2014).

The activity of matrix metalloproteinase (MMP)-8 lateral-flow POC immunotests is a commercially available, practical, convenient, and inexpensive test that takes about 5 min and claimed to detect, predict, and monitor the course and treatment of periodontitis (Hernandez et al. 2012; Heikkinen et al. 2016; Rathnayake et al. 2017). It is considered among the few tests where a biomarker can identify disease activity, predict progression, and monitor the response to periodontal treatment (Raisanen et al. 2019).

7.1.2 Lab-on-a-Chip Methods

These are newer generation of POC technology that incorporates sampling, sample preparation, detection, and data analysis all in one small device. This technology aims to measure multiple biomarkers in a small biofluid sample but it is yet to be developed.

7.1.3 Proteomic Analysis

Proteomics directly studies the proteins that are key functional components of biochemical systems and describes the large-scale study of the entire complement of proteins expressed by a genome and present in a cell, tissue, biofluids, or organism (Aebersold et al. 2000). The word "proteome" was introduced by Wilkins et al. (1996) as a combination of two words, "protein" and "genome". The proteome is the protein complement of the genome and proteomics is the analysis of the portion of the genome that is expressed. The human proteome is estimated to contain more than 20,000 proteins, excluding possible isoforms. There are two strategies for proteomic applications: discovery (qualification) and quantification, mostly as the first and second step. After surface enhanced laser desorption/ionisation-time-of-flight mass spectrometry was invented, mass spectral fingerprints of proteins were detected basing on their molecular weight rather than their sequence identity within the context of qualitative proteomics. This earlier technology was successfully applied to GCF proteome analysis, but solely it cannot reveal the identity of proteins or their functions. The advancement of analytical proteomic platforms came with the combined use of in-gel digestion along with their extensive separation and enhanced spectral analysis (Bostanci and Belibasakis 2018).

Later on, quantitative proteomics were applied to GCF samples. Proteomics has the potential to produce low-cost POC devices (Wignarajah et al. 2015; Koboniwa et al. 2016). However, one of the major challenges in identification and quantification of the GCF or salivary proteome is the dynamic range of protein concentrations often spanning several orders of magnitude. There is a risk of being masked for the proteins that have the lowest relative amounts in the complex mixture. Immune depletion of the abundant proteins such as albumin may help unmasking those low-abundance proteins, but at the same time this may cause removal of several others structurally bound to them. Furthermore, pre-analytical steps such as sample elution as well as mathematical analysis may also affect the findings.

Saliva has been used as a biofluid for proteomics analysis and more than 3000 proteins have been identified for disease (Zhang et al. 2016). Moreover, evidence suggests that proteomics facilitate the identification of GCF biochemical markers in patients with periodontal disease (Bostanci et al. 2010; Bostanci and Bao 2017; Bostanci and Belibasakis 2018; Khurshid et al. 2017). Today, proteomics are used for discovering and identifying GCF biomarkers with matrix-assisted laser desorption/ionisation time-of-flight mass spectrometry (MALDI-TOF MS), liquid chromatography (LC) coupled with tandem mass spectrometry (MS/MS) (LC-MS/MS) (Fig. 7.2).

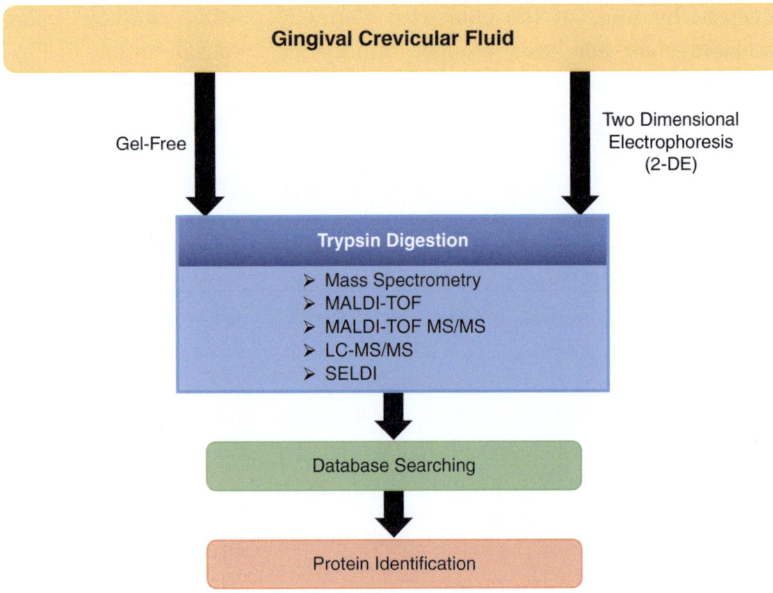

Fig. 7.2 Proteomic analysis techniques used for GCF samples

7.1.4 Mass Spectrometry (MS)

Recent technological developments in proteomics and mass spectrometry have provided promising methods and valuable data for discovery of biomarkers for various diseases including periodontitis. Collection method of GCF samples and handling procedures can have a significant effect on the proteome (Lee et al. 2010). It is recommended to store the samples at the coldest freezer possible, particularly for longer storage periods. Preiano et al. (2014, 2018) reported that samples could be stored stabile at −80 °C for months.

Mass spectrometry based on quantitative proteomics: Proteins can be labelled metabolically with heavy or light isotope-containing growth media, and derivatisation can occur following proteolytic digestion using isotopically distinct chemical labels or isobaric tags (Zhu et al. 2018; Wright 2018; Yang et al. 2017). Other "label free" quantitation techniques eliminate labelling and instead rely on advanced software analysis. These methods measure the relative concentrations of peptide analytes within two or more samples. Conversely, absolute quantitation techniques use internal standard peptides that have been prepared synthetically for selected reaction monitoring (SRM) or multiple reaction monitoring (MRM) analysis and are gaining more popularity (Tsuchida et al. 2019). MRM technique can be combined with a quantitative MS technique involving stable isotype labelling by amino acids in cell culture (SILAC). Stable isotype labelling with SILAC experiments can quantify proteins and peptides accurately (Terzi and Cambridge 2017; Dittmar and Selbach 2015).

7.1.5 Shotgun Proteomics

This is an alternative approach that involves enzymatic digestion of whole proteins into small peptide fragments with uniform characteristics that are analysed directly by LC-MS/MS (Ogita et al. 2015; Tsuchida et al. 2012). Various proteomic analysis methods including MALDI-TOF/MS, gas chromatography MS (GC/MS), and LC/MS are being increasingly preferred in studies searching for biomarkers for periodontal diseases. MS allows not only identification but also quantification of as many as 317 proteins in GCF samples (Batschkus et al. 2017). In the near future, glycomics may also be applied to the study of GCF using MS.

7.1.6 Gel Electrophoresis

Gel electrophoresis is a method for separation and analysis of macromolecules and their fragments, based on their size and electrical charge. Gingival tissue samples can be analysed using this technique.

7.1.7 Genetics and Periodontal Diagnosis

Periodontal diseases particularly periodontitis have genetic susceptibility component. This statement is mainly based on the fact that not all individuals with similar amounts of contents of microbial dental plaque develop periodontal disease with similar extent and severity. No doubt, like many other chronic diseases, genetic factors are very important in the development of periodontitis, but they can only act as risk factors when challenged by extrinsic aetiological factors and physical irritants. Genetic polymorphisms are likely to contribute to the genetic susceptibility, but single nucleotide polymorphisms (SNPs) of DNA are not easily identified, particularly in multifactorial diseases like periodontitis. As a definition, an SNP has to occur in at least 1% of a given population, while individual mutations, not fixed in the population, are referred to as single nucleotide variations (SNVs) (Lindroth and Park 2013). Some SNPs alter gene expression levels that may affect host response against the microbial attacks from the dental plaque. These genes may be related with receptors or sensors in cell surfaces, or with cytokines and chemokines acting in the immune, inflammatory response to the dental biofilm. Although, some connections between genetic variation and periodontitis at some loci have been suggested, their penetrance remains elusive. It is challenging to elucidate the genetic background, as genetic polymorphisms that affect susceptibility are solely not deterministic for disease onset or progression. At present, specific candidate genes of susceptibility are unknown and the connection between SNPs and periodontitis is not always strong because of great variability within populations and defined or undefined subtypes of periodontitis.

Several genetic polymorphisms have been studied for possible association with periodontitis so far (Kinane and Hart 2003; Vijayalakshmi et al. 2010) failing to provide strong diagnostic or prognostic markers to identify patients within the general population that have high risk for periodontal disease. In a comprehensive study, Demmer et al. (2008) analysed the whole genome to show the differential gene expression of healthy and diseased periodontal sites and demonstrated several dysregulated genes in disease compared to health. However, this data could not be implemented in clinical diagnostic practice. On the other hand, it may be concluded that investigation of the relationship between genetics and periodontal disease progression helps to identify biomarkers with a potential diagnostic value (Giannobile 2012; Taba et al. 2012). As such, genome-wide association studies (GWAS) have identified novel genes for susceptibility for periodontitis (Schaefer et al. 2010; Divaris et al. 2013). The mechanisms how the identified susceptibility genes influence the pathogenesis of periodontitis are not clarified yet, but these studies open up new pathways for diagnostic approaches.

Salivary genome analysis indicated that 70% of it is human and 30% is microbial DNAs (Zhang et al. 2016). Although the approximate salivary mean total DNA is about 10 times lower than that of the circulation, 72–96% of salivary samples can be genotyped. Saliva samples are convenient for long-term storage for genomic analysis. Moreover, its quality and purity have been reported to be comparable to that of the blood (Wang et al. 2017). Salivary genetic and epigenetic analysis has been suggested to provide gene-transcription profiles that could reflect abnormal pathological genetic processes (Zhang et al. 2016).

7.1.8 Epigenetics

Epigenetics refers to the layers of chemical modifications on the DNA and its associated proteins that regulate gene expression and is described as changes in patterns of gene expression, which do not involve changes in the DNA sequence. These modifications are either erased or established depending on the environmental response leading to intracellular signalling. The environment may well have significant influences on genetics via epigenetics and the environment can cause heritable changes in living organisms. In a broader sense, normal differentiation, neoplastic changes, and changes caused by infections and inflammation are all forms of epigenetic modification (Benakanakere et al. 2019). Epigenetics has been linked to many diseases including cancer and inflammation and also to physiological states such as ageing. It is rather new in the field of periodontal disease research, but may well provide explanation for the higher prevalence of periodontitis in the elderly population.

One characteristic feature of the oral mucosa is to be continuously exposed to pathogens and commensal microorganisms. Thus, the cells of the gingiva must differentiate pathogens from commensals and instigate inflammatory responses to the former but not the latter. The persistent inflammation in the periodontium leads to constant cellular death and turnover leading to tissue regeneration process that could invoke specific epigenetic modifications resulting in a different phenotype. Studies have also shown that extrinsic environmental factors, growth factors and hormones that regulate differentiation, can cause epigenetic modifications (Cortessis et al. 2012). Evidence shows that a lifestyle of smoking, food intake, lack of exercise, and use of drugs strongly influences the epigenetic pattern and predisposes to most conditions that lead to human disease (Alegria-Torres et al. 2011). Chronic periodontitis invokes a high turnover of cells in the gingiva such as epithelial cells, fibroblasts, and bone forming cells necessary to replace cells lost due to cellular apoptosis (Stathopoulou et al. 2009). Any defect in these proliferating cells can lead to an aberrant cellular response that in turn leads to a variegated phenotype. High levels of cellular turnover and change in microbiota (pathogen vs. commensals) in the host may create discriminatory pressure in certain lesions leading to patches of epigenetic reprogramming (Benakanakere et al. 2019). Periodontitis is characterised by its variable subject and site-based susceptibility. It is possible that the epigenetic changes may occur at a particular region or there may be widespread changes in the epigenetic factors affecting most of the teeth in an individual. This high site-specificity may be epigenetically altered in their inflammatory responsiveness. To help explain this phenomenon, Benakanakere et al. (2019) coined the term "Periodontal Mosaicism" for this variegated phenotype in periodontitis and defined it as epigenetic variation in the gingiva leading to variation in disease susceptibility. Although epigenetic studies in periodontitis are limited, gingival cells have been suggested to have the ability to respond to environmental factors in attaining different phenotypes (Gomez et al. 2009). The inflammatory response in periodontitis is similar to other inflammatory diseases where upregulation of transcription factors like nuclear factor kappaB and chromatin changes occur that might induce epigenetic alterations (Bayarsaihan 2011), and more recently by Larsson (Larsson 2017), summarised epigenetic involvement in periodontal diseases.

7.1.9 Transcriptomics

Transcriptomics refers to total gene transcript analysis and it has been applied on periodontal tissue as well as peripheral blood cells. The human salivary transcriptome consists of mainly mRNA and microRNA (miRNA) (Zhang et al. 2016). Salivary mRNAs, as well as endogenous miRNAs, are protected from ribonucleases by exosomes in the saliva and are therefore resistant to degradation (Yoshizawa and Wong 2013).

7.1.10 Metabolomics

Metabolites are cellular products produced as a result of physiological cellular functions such as gene transcription, mRNA translation, protein synthesis, and metabolic enzymatic reactions. The comprehensive identification, quantification, and analysis of these metabolites are known as "metabolomics" (Washio and Takahashi 2016). The techniques such as capillary electrophoresis and a time-of-flight mass spectrometer allow detection of numerous metabolites in a small amount of biological sample. Such investigations are likely to provide researchers and clinicians valuable information on the diagnosis of oral diseases. Hence, metabolomics is regarded as a promising technology for discovering biomarkers, monitoring oral health status, and guiding clinicians in treatment planning and monitoring their patients.

7.2 Microbiological Laboratory Analyses

Microorganisms or their toxins and products can be detected by different methods (Fig. 7.3). Direct microscopic investigation, culturing live bacteria, DNA probes, checkerboard DNA–DNA hybridisation, and polymerase chain reaction (PCR) are the major microbiological techniques. Immunologic techniques can also be used for indirect detection of microorganisms. These immunologic techniques are direct and indirect immunofluorescence assay (IFA), flow cytometry, ELISA, membrane assays, and latex agglutination (Belibasakis et al. 2019). There are available chair-side-tests for detection of major periodontal pathogens (Arweiler et al. 2019).

7.2.1 Culture Technique

Culturing microorganisms allows detection and quantification of all cultivable bacterial species and considered as the gold standard in microbiological testing. It is also convenient to detect superinfecting organisms such as Candida species, staphylococci, enterococci, etc. Moreover, antibiotic susceptibility testing can only be applied to cultivated microorganisms. Only the live bacteria can be cultivated and this can be considered as a drawback since remnants or cellular particles of some microorganisms can also trigger host response and activate pathogenic mechanisms. On the other hand, discriminating live bacteria may provide extremely valuable information on the pathogenesis as well as treatment of an infectious disease. The other pitfalls of the culture technique are the technical difficulty of cultivating anaerobic bacteria (sampling, storage, transfer of the samples), the need for special laboratory equipment, experienced staff, and finally being time-consuming.

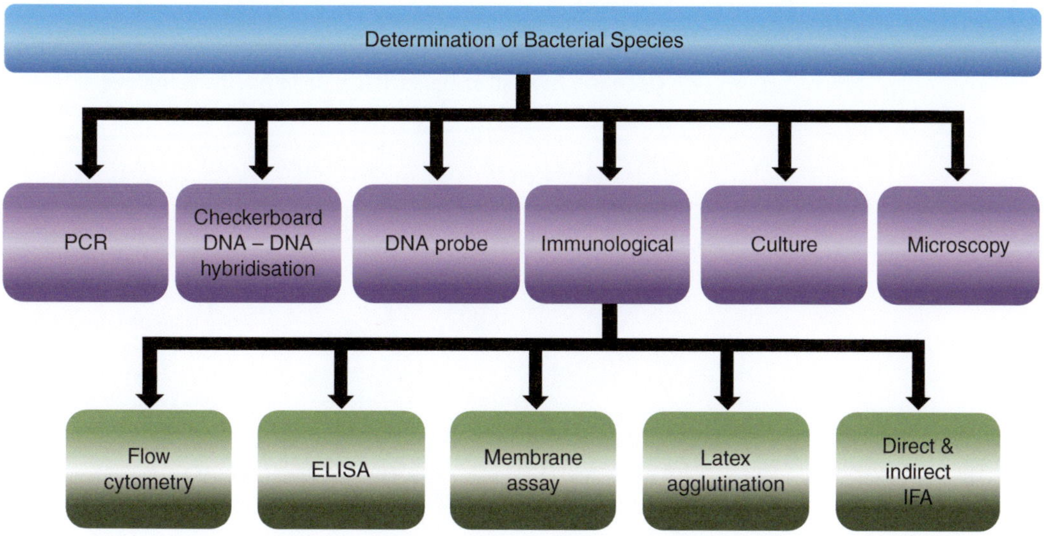

Fig. 7.3 Laboratory techniques available for microbiological investigation

7.2.2 Polymerase Chain Reaction (PCR)

This technique can overcome the disadvantages of the culture technique and can be used either for qualitative or quantitative purposes. Qualitative methods include PCR based and enzymatic methods. Real-time PCR (RT-PCR) is used for measuring the amount of DNA and it can be used for both qualitative and quantitative purposes (Fig. 7.4). Saliva and GCF samples can also be analysed for microbiological content by RT-PCR.

7.2.3 Checkerboard DNA–DNA Hybridisation

This microbiological analysis technique was used by Socransky et al. (1994). The sensitivity and specificity of whole genomic probes have been described by Gunaratnam et al. (1992) and a comparison between checkerboard hybridisation and culture in the identification of subgingival microbiota has been reported (Papapanou et al. 1997).

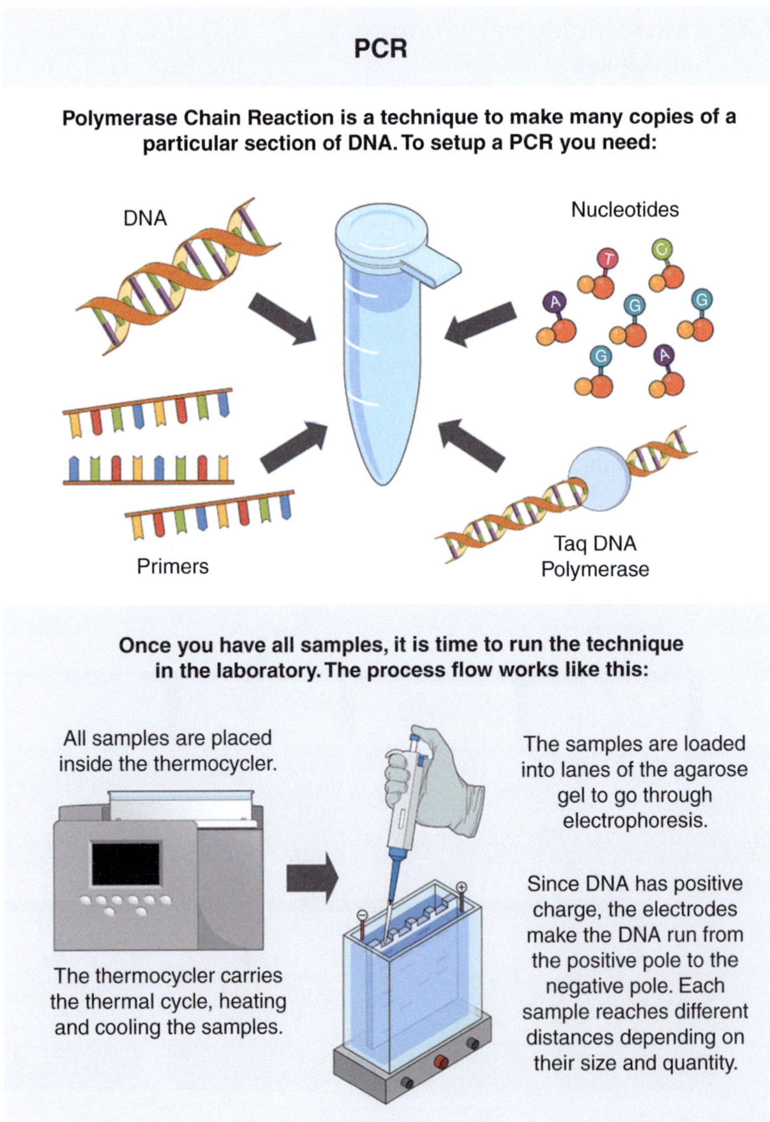

Fig. 7.4 Basic principles of PCR

7.3 Conclusion

Unravelling the quantitative changes of host and bacteria-derived GCF proteins will improve the knowledge on GCF protein composition and clarify specific alterations occurring in protein content that may be used as biomarkers for periodontal disease. There is still a long way to go; however, technological developments together with the curiosity and passion of researchers will eventually make it come true! Particularly prospective biomarkers are highly required.

References

Aebersold R, Rist B, Gygi SP. Quantitative proteome analysis: methods and applications. Ann N Y Acad Sci. 2000;919:33–47.

Alegria-Torres JA, Baccarelli A, Bollati V. Epigenetics and lifestyle. Epigenomics. 2011;3:267–77.

Arweiler NB, Marx VK, Laugisch O, Sculean A, Auschill TM. Clinical evaluation of a newly developed chair side test to determine periodontal pathogens. J Periodontol. 2019; https://doi.org/10.1002/JPER.19-0180. [Epub ahead of print]

Batschkus S, Cingoez G, Urlaub H, Miosge N, Kirschneck C, Meyer-Marcotty P, Lenz C. A new albumin-depletion strategy improves proteomic research of gingival crevicular fluid from periodontitis patients. Clin Oral Investig. 2017;22:1375–84.

Bayarsaihan D. Epigenetic mechanisms in inflammation. J Dent Res. 2011;90:9–17.

Belibasakis GN, Bostanci N, Marsh PD, Zaura E. Applications of the oral microbiome in personalised dentistry. Arch Oral Biol. 2019;104:7–12.

Benakanakere M, Finoti L, Palioto DB, Teixeira HS, Kinane DF. Epigenetics, inflammation and periodontal disease. Curr Oral Health Rep. 2019;6:37–46.

Bostanci N, Heywood W, Mills K, Parkar M, Nibali L, Donos N. Application of label-free absolute quantitative proteomics in human gingival crevicular fluid by LC/MSE (gingival exudatome). J Proteome Res. 2010;9:2191–9.

Bostanci N, Bao K. Contribution of proteomics to our understanding of periodontal inflammation. Proteomics. 2017;17:1500518.

Bostanci N, Belibasakis GN. Gingival crevicular fluid and its immune mediators in the proteomic era. Periodontol 2000. 2018;76:68–84.

Christodoulides N, Floriano PN, Miller CS, et al. Lab-on-a-chip methods for point-of-care measurements of salivary biomarkers of periodontitis. Ann N Y Acad Sci. 2007;1098:411–28.

Cortessis VK, Thomas DC, Levine AJ, Breton CV, Mack TM, Siegmund KD, et al. Environmental epigenetics: prospects for studying epigenetic mediation of exposure-response relationships. Hum Genet. 2012;131:1565–89.

Demmer RT, Behle JH, Wolf DL, et al. Transcriptomes in healthy and diseased gingival tissues. J Periodontol. 2008;79:2112–24.

Dittmar G, Selbach M. SILAC for biomarker discovery. Proteomics Clin Appl. 2015;9:301–6.

Divaris K, Monda KL, North KE, Olshan AF, Reynolds LM, Hsueh WC, et al. Exploring the genetic basis of chronic periodontitis: a genome-wide association study. Hum Mol Genet. 2013;22:2312–24.

Giannobile WV. Salivary diagnostics for periodontal diseases. JADA. 2012;143(Suppl.10):6s–11s.

Gomez RS, Dutra WO, Moreira PR. Epigenetics and periodontal disease: future perspectives. Inflamm Res. 2009;58:625–9.

Gunaratnam M, Smith GLF, Socransky SS, Smith CM, Haffajee AD. Enumeration of subgingival species on primary isolation plates using colony lifts. Oral Microbiol Immunol. 1992;7:14–8.

Heikkinen AM, Nwhator SO, Rathnayake N, Mantyla P, Vatanen P, Sorsa T. Pilot study on oral health status as assessed by an active matrix metalloproteinase-8 chairside mouthrinse test in adolescents. J Periodontol. 2016;87:36–40.

Hernandez M, Vernal R, Sorsa T, Tervahartiala T, Mantyla P, Gamonal J. The role of immune-inflammatory response in the pathogenesis of chronic periodontitis and development of chair-side point-of-care diagnostics. In: Buduneli N, editor. Pathogenesis and treatment of periodontitis. Pp: InTech Publishing Co.; 2012. p. 33–54.

Jaedicke KM, Preshaw PM, Taylor JJ. Salivary cytokines as diagnostic biomarkers of periodontal diseases. Periodontol 2000. 2016;70:164–83.

Kaczor-Urbanowicz KE, Carreras-Presas CM, Aro K, Tu M, Garcia-Godoy F, Wong DTW. Saliva diagnostics-current views and directions. Exp Biol Med. 2016;242:459–72.

Kinane DF, Hart TC. Genes and gene polymorphisms associated with periodontal disease. Crit Rev Oral Biol Med. 2003;14:430–49.

Koboniwa M, Sakanaka A, Hashino E, Bamba T, Fukusaki E, Amano A. Prediction of periodontal inflammation via metabolic profiling of saliva. J Dent Res. 2016;95:1381–6.

Khurshid Z, Mali M, Naseem M, Najeeb S, Zafar MS. Human gingival crevicular fluids (GCF) proteomics: an overview. Dent J. 2017;5:12.

Larsson L. Current concepts of epigenetics and its role in periodontitis. Curr Oral Health Rep. 2017;4:286–93.

Lee DH, Kim JW, Jeon SY, Park BK, Han BG. Proteomic analysis of the effect of storage temperature on human serum. Ann Clin Lab Sci. 2010;40:61–70.

Lindroth AM, Park YJ. Epigenetic biomarkers: a step forward for understanding periodontitis. J Periodontal Implant Sci. 2013;43:111–20.

Lorenzo-Poso AI, Perez-Sayans M, Bravo SB, Lopez-Jornet P, Garcia-Vence M, Alonso-Sampedro M,

Carballo J. Protein-based salivary profiles as novel biomarkers for oral diseases. Dis Markers. 2018;2018:6141845.

Miller CS, Foley JD, Bailey AL, Campell CL, Humphries RL, Christodoulides N, et al. Current developments in salivary diagnostics. Biomark Med. 2010;4:171–89.

Ogawa Y, Miura Y, Harazono A, et al. Proteomic analysis of two types of exosomes in human whole saliva. Biol Pharm Bull. 2011;34:13–23.

Ogita M, Tsuchida S, Aoki A, Satoh M, Kado S, Sawabe M, Nanbara H, Kobayashi H, Takeuchi Y, et al. Increased cell proliferation and differential protein expression induced by low-level Er:YAG laser irradiation in human gingival fibroblasts: proteomic analysis. Lasers Med Sci. 2015;30:1855–66.

Papapanou PN, Madianos PN, Dahlen G, Sandros J. "Checkerboard" versus culture: a comparison between two methods for identification of subgingival microbiota. Eur J Oral Sci. 1997;105:389–96.

Preiano M, Falcone D, Maggisano G, Montalcini T, Navarra M, Paduano S, Savino R, Terracciano R. Assessment of pre-analytical and analytical variables affecting peptidome profiling of gingival crevicular fluid by MALDI-TOF mass spectrometry. Clin Chim Acta. 2014;437:120–8.

Preiano M, Maggisano G, Murfuni MS, Villella C, Pelaia C, Montalcini T, Lombardo N, Pelaia G, Savino R, Terracciano R. An analytical method for assessing optimal storage conditions of gingival crevicular fluid and disclosing a peptide biomarker signature of gingivitis by MALDI-TOF MS. Proteomics Clin Appl. 2018;12:1800005.

Raisanen IT, Sorsa T, van der Schoor GJ, et al. Active matrix metalloproteinase-8 point-of-care (PoC/Chairside mouthrinse test vs. bleeding on probing in diagnosing subclinical periodontitis in adolescents). Diagnostics (Basel). 2019;9(1):34.

Rathnayake N, Gieselmann DR, Heikkinen AM, Tervahartiala T, Sorsa T. Salivary diagnostic point-of-care diagnostics of MMP-8 in dentistry and medicine. Diagnostics (Basel). 2017;7(1):E7.

Sackman EK, Fulton AL, Beebe DJ. The present and future role of biofluidics in biomedical research. Nature. 2014;507:181–9.

Schaefer AS, richter GM, Nothnagel M, Manke T, Dommisch H, Jacobs G, et al. A genome-wide association study identifies GLT6D1 as a susceptibility locus for periodontitis. Hum Mol Genet. 2010;19:553–62.

Sexton WM, Lin Y, Kryscio RJ, Dawson DR 3rd, Ebersole JL, Miller CS. Salivary biomarkers of periodontal disease in response to treatment. J Clin Periodontol. 2011;38:434–41.

Socransky SS, Smith C, Martin L, Paster BJ, Dewhirst FE, Levin AE. "Checkerboard" DNA-DNA hybridisation. BioTechniques. 1994;17:788–92.

Spielmann N, Wong DT. Saliva: diagnostics and therapeutic perspectives. Oral Dis. 2011;17:345–54.

Stathopoulou PG, Benakanakere MR, Galicia JC, Kinane DF. The host cytokine response to Porphyromonas gingivalis is modified by gingipains. Oral Microbiol Immunol. 2009;24:11–7.

Taba M, Souza SL, Mariguela VC. Periodontal disease: a genetic perspective. Braz Oral Res. 2012;26(Suppl. 1):32–8.

Terzi F, Cambridge S. An overview of advanced SILAC-labelling strategies for quantitative proteomics. Methods Enzymol. 2017;585:29–47.

Tsuchida S, Satoh M, Umemura H, Sogawa K, Kawashima Y, Kado S, Sawai S, Nishimura M, Kodera Y, Matsushita K, Nomura F. Proteomic analysis of gingival crevicular fluid for discovery of novel periodontal disease markers. Proteomics. 2012;12:2190–202.

Tsuchida S, Satoh M, Takiwaki M, Nomura F. Current status of proteomic technologies for discovering and identifying gingival crevicular fluid biomarkers for periodontal disease. Int J Mol Sci. 2019;20:86.

Vijayalakshmi R, Geetha A, Ramakrishnan T, Emmadi P. Genetic polymorphisms in periodontal diseases: an overview. Indian J Dental Research. 2010;21:568–74.

Wang CC, Huang RP, Sommer M, Lisoukov H, Huang R, Lin Y, Miller T, Burke J. Array-based multiplexed screening and quantitation of human cytokines and chemokines. J Proteome Res. 2002;1:337–43.

Wang X, Kaczor-Urbanowicz KE, Wong DTW. Salivary biomarkers in cancer detection. Med Oncol. 2017;34:7.

Washio J, Takahashi N. Metabolomic studies of oral biofilm. Oral cancer and beyond. Int J Mol Sci. 2016;17:870.

Wassall RR, Preshaw PM. Clinical and technical considerations in the analysis of gingival crevicular fluid. Periodontol 2000. 2016;70:65–79.

Wignarajah S, Sualfan GA, Bizzaro S, Bikker FJ, Kaman WE, Zourob M. Colorimetric assay for the detection of typical biomarkers for periodontitis using a magnetic nanoparticle biosensor. Anal Chem. 2015;87:12161–8.

Wilkins MR, Pasquali C, Appel RD, et al. From proteins to proteomes: large scale protein identification by two-dimensional electrophoresis and amino acid analysis. Biotechnology (NY). 1996;14:61–5.

Wright MH. Chemical proteomics of host-microbe interactions. Proteomics. 2018;18:e1700333.

Yang Y, Fonovic M, Verhelst SH. Cleavable linkers in chemical proteomics applications. Methods Mol Biol. 2017;1491:185–203.

Yoshizawa JM, Wong DT. Salivary microRNAs and oral cancer detection. Methods Mol Biol. 2013;936:313–24.

Zhang Y, Sun J, Lin CC, Abemayor E, Wang MB, Wong DT. The emerging landscape of salivary diagnostics. Periodontol 2000. 2016;70:38–52.

Zhu H, Tamura T, Hamachi I. Chemical proteomics for subcellular proteome analysis. Curr Opin Chem Biol. 2018;48:1–7.

Biomarkers in Periodontal Disease and Systemic Health Intersection

8

Studies published particularly in the last two decades indicated that there is a close relationship between oral and general health and a two-way interaction is likely to exist in some instances, particularly in diabetes (Kinane and Chestnutt 1997). Microbial dental plaque or oral biofilm is the primary cause of periodontal diseases and more than 700 different bacterial species have been identified in the oral cavity so far (Dewhirst et al. 2010). Total bacterial count in 1 ml of saliva can reach very high numbers like 10^8–10^9 (Larsen and Fiehn 2017). These bacteria themselves or their toxins can trigger host immune response creating an inflammatory reaction in the periodontal tissues. This inflammation, although designed to protect the host, may be responsible for the major part of the tissue destruction observed in periodontitis.

Periodontitis is chronic and infectious in nature and characterised by irreversible loss of periodontal attachment and alveolar bone. Apart from the biofilm, environmental factors such as smoking and systemic diseases such as diabetes mellitus have significant impact on the extent and severity of periodontitis. Moreover, there are genetic risk factors affecting the host inflammatory response, connective tissue, and bone metabolism that may change the course and clinical signs of periodontitis (Loos et al. 2015). Numerous cytokines, enzymes, and other inflammatory mediators deriving from neutrophils, monocytes, macrophages, T-cells, B-cells, or resident cells such as fibroblasts, keratinocytes, and endothelial cells are all components of the extensive orchestra in play in periodontal tissue destruction.

Diagnosis of periodontal diseases mainly relies on the clinical signs and symptoms in terms of probing depth, clinical attachment level, bleeding on probing, oral hygiene level, and radiographic findings. However, these clinical periodontal parameters provide information about the past; that is, they are post-symptomatic and do neither clarify the current situation nor predict the prognosis. Furthermore, clinical periodontal indices are subjective and have low sensitivity and low specificity. The standard error of clinical periodontal measurements with manual periodontal probes is roughly ± 1 mm. These facts have urged the search for biomarkers that will objectively and quantitatively assess the extent and severity of periodontal disease. Why do we need to diagnose? Why is the accurate diagnosis of periodontal disease important? We need reliable and reproducible measures for discrimination of not only disease from health but also active sites from sites in remission in order to appropriately tailor our treatment for the individual clinical conditions. Another great challenge is to find predictive biomarkers for periodontal tissue destruction and to make individually tailored treatment protocols.

During the last 50 years, new technologies have been introduced in the field of periodontics.

N. Buduneli, *Biomarkers in Periodontal Health and Disease*,
https://doi.org/10.1007/978-3-030-37317-7_8

Pressure sensitive probes, electronic patient record systems, voice-activated charting systems, new imaging techniques such as subtraction radiography and cone-beam tomography are among those novel technologies. However, they failed to provide a real conceptual change in periodontal diagnostics. Biomarkers may fulfil these prerequisites and therefore the search for valid biomarkers has been the topic of interest for many years now.

On the other hand, various systemic diseases or health problems may affect the course of periodontal diseases or vice versa. Thus, markers in blood circulation and/or saliva have a potential to provide information on the possible link between oral and systemic health. This review focuses on salivary and/or serum biomarkers that may help to diagnose periodontal diseases and may also assist in explaining pathogenic mechanisms and the interaction mechanisms between periodontal diseases and some systemic diseases.

8.1 What Is a Biomarker?

A biomarker can be defined as an objective indication of disease status observed from outside the patient that can be measured accurately and reproducibly. A measurable biomarker can act as a reliable indicator of the biological process and it can be applied to diagnosis, staging, and also prognosis of a certain disease. An ideal biomarker should be safe and easy to measure, it should change with treatment, thus ideally reflect the patient's response to treatment. It must be highly sensitive, specific, and cost-effective for use in follow-up and be consistent across gender and ethnic groups. Preferentially, an ideal biomarker should be appropriate for chair-side use with 1-stage or 2-stage procedure.

8.2 Systemic Biomarkers in Saliva

Saliva is a biofluid that is readily available, can be obtained in a non-invasive way, i.e., minor inconvenience to the patient. Its collection does not require any specific instrument or personnel. Saliva samples can be unstimulated or stimulated and can be whole saliva or sampled from a specific salivary gland. Saliva is regarded as a "mirror of the body". Ongoing studies focus on possible salivary diagnostic tests not only for oral diseases but also for systemic diseases such as diabetes, myocardial infarction, or even pancreatic cancer (Floriano et al. 2009; Miller et al. 2014). The flow as well as content of saliva is affected by the circadian rhythm. Moreover, its volume can exhibit individual variability depending on the age, systemic health state, smoking habits of the person, or drugs used, etc. This fact makes the interpretation of the salivary data problematic.

More than 2000 proteins have been identified so far in human salivary samples (Grassl et al. 2016). Among the most investigated candidate salivary biomarkers for periodontal diseases are inflammatory cytokines, destructive enzymes, and antibodies. A promising candidate biomarker is salivary matrix metalloproteinase-8 (MMP-8) level and a chair-side diagnostic test has been stated to reliably diagnose and monitor the prognosis of periodontitis (Heikkenen et al. 2016). Several cross-sectional studies indicated significant positive correlations between clinical periodontal parameters and salivary MMP-8 levels (Miller et al. 2006; Ramseier et al. 2009; Costa et al. 2010; Gursoy et al. 2010; Kinney et al. 2011). Recently, a meta-analysis indicated that periodontitis patients exhibited significantly higher salivary MMP-8 levels compared to the periodontally healthy counterparts (Zhang et al. 2018). Moreover, non-surgical periodontal treatment has been reported to provide significant reductions in salivary MMP-8 levels suggesting that it can be indicative of the response to therapy (Sexton et al. 2011).

Numerous studies documented similar significant correlations between salivary levels of pro-inflammatory cytokines such as interleukin-1beta (IL-ß), IL-6, tumour necrosis factor-alpha (TNF-α), receptor activator of nuclear factor kappaB ligand (RANKL), and osteoprotegerin (OPG) and clinical periodontal findings (Miller et al. 2006; Costa et al. 2010; Buduneli et al. 2008;

Gursoy et al. 2011). Recently, salivary levels of IL-1ß and hepatocyte growth factor (HGF) were reported to be the most robust biomarkers for periodontal diseases (Jaedicke et al. 2016). HGF is produced by periodontal ligament cells and fibroblasts and enhances production of MMPs, may drive apical migration of epithelial cells in periodontitis. Consistent data from cross-sectional studies as well as few longitudinal studies suggest its salivary level as a potential biomarker for periodontitis (Jaedicke et al. 2016).

On the other hand, various oxidative stress markers for lipid peroxidation, protein oxidation, and DNA damage can be detected in saliva samples in relation with periodontal health. Salivary oxidative stress markers have been suggested to have the potential for diagnosis and monitoring of periodontal diseases (Baltacıoğlu et al. 2014; Baňasová et al. 2015; Villa-Correa et al. 2015). Furthermore, significant positive correlation between salivary total antioxidant capacity (TAC) and periodontal disease was reported by Novakovic et al. (Novakovic et al. 2014). Accordingly, salivary melatonin levels showed positive correlation with periodontal inflammation and decreased following periodontal treatment (Bertl et al. 2013). Oxidative stress markers in saliva samples seem to be derived from local events; however, it is not clear yet whether an increase in their local production or a decrease in their feedback in terms of antioxidants or both mechanisms cause the net effect. Thus, further studies are required to better clarify their possible role in periodontal diagnostics.

8.3 Systemic Biomarkers in Circulation

Serum or plasma samples can be obtained from a venous blood sample. Periodontal diseases can have manifestations in the circulation and various systemic diseases/states can have significant effects on periodontal disease progression.

Upon a stimulus from an inflammatory agent, host inflammatory cells release cytokines such as interleukin (IL)-1, IL-6, tumour necrosis-alpha (TNF-α), and interferon-gamma (IFN-γ), which then stimulate secretion of acute phase reactants by the liver. C-reactive protein (CRP) is the major acute phase reactant. Findings of cross-sectional studies were re-evaluated in a meta-analysis and the authors concluded that the plasma CRP concentration is elevated in patients with periodontal disease compared to those with clinically healthy periodontium (Paraskevas et al. 2008). The authors documented strong evidence for elevated CRP in patients with periodontal disease and modest evidence for a decrease in CRP levels following non-surgical periodontal treatment. However, this is also likely to be related with comorbidities and confounders such as bacteria or virus infections not affecting periodontal tissues. A recent randomised clinical trial showed for the first time that non-surgical periodontal treatment decreased plasma CRP, IL-6, and fibrinogen levels in patients with severe periodontitis and severe non-responsive arterial hypertension under medical treatment (Vidal et al. 2009). A large study involving 4830 Scottish adults reported that those with poor oral hygiene had higher concentrations of CRP and fibrinogen (de Oliveira et al. 2010). Only a few longitudinal studies investigating possible relationship between periodontal disease and systemic CRP levels have been published so far. Positive correlation was found between clinical periodontal disease findings and CRP in a longitudinal study involving 11,162 Japanese men (Yoshii et al. 2009). There are also studies reporting higher levels of the other acute phase reactants such as IL-18 and fibrinogen in patients with periodontal diseases (Buhlin et al. 2009). The available literature on the topic suggests that periodontal diseases cause a low-grade systemic inflammation. A systematic review and meta-analysis of randomised controlled trials investigating effects of anti-infective periodontal treatment on CRP reported a modest short-term reduction in CRP levels (Demmer et al. 2013).

Pentraxins (PTXs) are a superfamily of multi-functional proteins, and PTX-3 behaves as an acute phase protein since its blood levels, which are low in normal conditions, increase rapidly and dramatically during inflammatory and infectious conditions and correlate with the severity of the acute condition (Garlanda et al. 2009). PTX-3 is produced by IL-1 stimulation, TNF-α, or oxidised-low-density lipoprotein, which are factors known to be prominent in periodontal diseases. Salivary and serum levels of PTX-3 have been investigated comparatively in patients with periodontitis and periodontally healthy individuals and were found to be correlated with clinical periodontal parameters (Gümüş et al. 2014). The authors concluded that its salivary concentrations might have a diagnostic potential for periodontal inflammation.

In a recent study comparing patients with or without chronic periodontitis, it was reported that higher serum resistin levels found in patients with chronic periodontitis suggest that its serum levels may be used as a surrogate marker to identify subjects at risk for periodontitis or reflect comorbidity (Akram et al. 2017). Moreover, the authors stated that confounding systemic diseases such as diabetes, obesity, or rheumatoid arthritis did not affect the serum levels.

Antimicrobial peptides have a controlling role in both innate and acquired immune responses and its local dysregulation is implicated in the pathogenesis of periodontal disease. Systemic diseases such as diabetes and rheumatoid arthritis and environmental factors such as tobacco smoking also affect their expressions. A very recent systematic review concluded that antimicrobial peptides could be a possible mechanistic link between periodontal diseases and related systemic diseases (Li et al. 2018). However, the authors also pointed out the need for further clinical and in vitro studies to better clarify the issue.

8.4 Systemic Biomarkers in Association with Systemic Diseases

Periodontal diseases have been suggested to increase the risk of stroke, cardiovascular diseases, diabetes, respiratory diseases, adverse pregnancy outcomes, kidney diseases, etc. (Tsuchida et al. 2019).

Diabetes mellitus is one of the most common systemic diseases worldwide. It has significant consequences on immune response and wound healing that play critical roles in the pathogenesis as well as response to treatment of various diseases including periodontal diseases. Metabolic control of diabetes is the major factor that determines its systemic effects that is evaluated by the percentage of glycated haemoglobin A1c (HbA1c) in the circulation. Periodontal diseases negatively affect glycaemic control in diabetic patients, and treatment of periodontitis helps to improve the level of this biomarker (Hasuike et al. 2017). Kardeşler et al. (2010) reported that non-surgical periodontal treatment helped to improve the glycaemic control in patients with poorly controlled type 2 diabetes and severe periodontitis. The authors suggested that the decrease in serum levels of IL-6, TNF-α, CRP, and leptin together with the increase in adiponectin following non-surgical periodontal treatment might be a function of glycaemic control in patients with type 2 diabetes.

Glycated haemoglobin and glycated albumin are intermediate products involved in the nonenzymatic glycation reactions of blood proteins that finally change to advanced glycation end products. The glycated haemoglobin level (HbA1C) represents the mean glycaemic status over the previous 2–3 months and the glycated albumin level indicates the glycaemic condition during the last 2–3 weeks. Glycated albumin in GCF was suggested to be a marker associated with disease progression in diabetic patients (Koga and Kasayama 2010).

Obesity is another epidemic health problem and there is substantial evidence from in vivo and in vitro studies demonstrating a strong association between periodontitis and obesity (Akram et al. 2016). However, mechanisms in this interaction have not been explained yet. Serum leptin and IL-6 levels together with clinical periodontal measurements were compared between obese and non-obese individuals in a cross-sectional study (Buduneli et al. 2014). The authors reported that obese participants did not exhibit worse clinical periodontal findings, but suggested that increased serum leptin and IL-6 levels may be one explanation for the possible interaction between obesity and periodontal disease.

A recent systematic review and meta-analysis evaluating the efficacy of non-surgical periodontal treatment in the management of periodontitis in obese or non-obese patients reported inconsistent findings in serum pro-inflammatory cytokine levels (IL-1ß, IL-6, TNF-α, IFN-γ, leptin, adiponectin, and CRP) (Akram et al. 2016).

Rheumatoid arthritis is another chronic inflammatory disease, which has common pathogenic mechanisms with periodontitis and has been investigated in many clinical studies focusing on possible two-way interactions between these two common chronic diseases. Non-surgical periodontal treatment in patients with severe periodontitis and rheumatoid arthritis provided significant decrease in DAS28 scores but no significant changes in IL-1ß and TNF-α levels (Bıyıkoğlu et al. 2013) A recent systematic review evaluating effects of non-surgical periodontal treatment in patients with periodontitis and rheumatoid arthritis reported a clear decrease in DAS28 score and erythrocyte sedimentation rate, while other inflammatory parameters such as CRP, IL-6, and TNF-α showed a non-significant tendency to decrease (Sivestre et al. 2016).

Polycystic ovarian syndrome (PCOS) is a complex disease characterised by hyperandrogenism and chronic anovulation. The influence of PCOS in non-obese women on salivary and serum concentrations of TNF-α, TNF-α receptors, and IL-6 and a possible association of these pro-inflammatory cytokines with PCOS and gingivitis was sought in a cross-sectional study (Özçaka et al. 2012). It was concluded that PCOS and gingival inflammation might act synergistically on the pro-inflammatory cytokines; IL-6 and TNF-α. Thus, PCOS may have an impact on gingival inflammation or vice versa. The same group investigated salivary and serum MMP-9, myeloperoxidase, neutrophil elastase, MMP-9/tissue inhibitor of MMP-1 (TIMP-1) ratio in the same patient population and reported an association between PCOS and gingival inflammation as evidenced by neutrophilic enzyme levels (Akcalı et al. 2017a).

Thalassemia is considered as the most common genetic disorder worldwide, presenting major public health and social problems. Thalassemia major has been suggested to exacerbate the local inflammatory response as manifested in salivary MMP-8, MMP-9, TIMP-1 levels (Gümüş et al. 2016). Moreover, it was reported to be related with periodontal disease via dysregulation of lymphocytes and increased activation of osteoclasts through the alterations in salivary and serum levels of soluble RANKL, osteoprotegerin, a proliferation-inducing ligand, B-cell activating factor, IL-6, and IL-8 (Akcalı et al. 2015).

Periodontal diseases and systemic biomarkers have also been investigated in women with gestational diabetes (GDM), and salivary and serum levels of inflammatory markers (sRANKL, IL-8, B-cell activating factor, MMP-8) have been found to be increased in patients with GDM and gingivitis (Akcalı et al. 2017b; Gümüş et al. 2015).

8.5 Limitations of Systemic Biomarkers as Periodontal Diagnostics

Periodontal diseases have a complex and multifactorial nature, and are episodic. Moreover, the clinical periodontal outcomes are the result of the complex interactions between microbial factors, host response, genetic susceptibility factors, systemic diseases, and environmental factors. Therefore, it is not likely to find a single biomarker for diagnosis and/or monitoring of periodontal diseases. Focusing on various combinations of biomarkers may be a more realistic approach to explain their possible roles in periodontal disease pathogenesis and the interactions between systemic health and periodontal diseases.

8.6 Conclusion

Periodontal diseases are chronic, infectious, inflammatory, and multifactorial in nature. The primary aetiological agent is the microbial dental plaque. However, the net effects of destructive enzymes and inflammatory cytokines released from host cells upon stimulation by microbial plaque factors are the major causes of periodontal tissue destruction. On the other hand, periodontal diseases can cause systemic inflammation and various systemic diseases/states can affect the periodontal inflammation. Therefore, investigation of possible biomarkers may help to explain the pathogenic mechanisms and help to diagnose and monitor periodontal diseases. Such information may also help to develop individually tailored periodontal treatment strategies according to the individual patient's periodontal and systemic health state.

Currently available data on biomarkers for periodontal diagnostics are still at their infancy and the evidence is too restricted. There are major methodological problems in studies focusing on this issue, as is the case for many other topics in the research field of periodontology. Saliva sampling methods, detection techniques, clinical diagnostic criteria, and statistical handling of the data show great variation between the published studies. Future studies with standard methodology will make a great contribution to the issue. Sensitivity and specificity values of candidate biomarkers should always be reported and should be preferentially high.

Salivary IL-1ß level seems to be the most promising biomarker for inflammation-related part of periodontal disease, whereas MMP-8 is the strongest candidate for tissue destruction. PTX-3 seems to be prominent as an acute phase protein biomarker and HGF has a potential as an immune system component. However, future studies may focus on a panel of biomarkers instead of investigating a single parameter.

The classification of periodontal diseases has been changed very recently (Papapanou et al. 2018). Biomarkers have been suggested to be directly involved in the grading of periodontal disease progression (Tonetti et al. 2018). However, the limitation of the available data did not enable doing so. Systemic health of participants particularly the presence/absence of diabetes and its level of metabolic control must be definitely taken into consideration and relevant data must be reported in future studies. Smoking status of participants must be recorded and chemically validated, but smokers should not be excluded from particularly the intervention studies in order not to lose data. Future studies with large scale and long follow-ups involving periodontal interventions are warranted to better clarify the place of systemic biomarkers in periodontics.

References

Akcalı A, Kahraman-Çeneli S, Gümüş P, Buduneli N, Lappin DF, Özçaka Ö. The association between thalassemia major and periodontal health. J Periodontol. 2015;86(9):1047–57.

Akcalı A, Bostanci N, Özçaka Ö, et al. Gingival inflammation and salivary or serum granulocyte-secreted enzymes in patients with polycystic ovary syndrome. J Periodontol. 2017a;88(11):1145–52.

Akcalı A, Gümüş P, Özçaka Ö, et al. Proteolytic mediators in gestational diabetes mellitus and gingivitis. J Periodontol. 2017b;88(3):289–97.

Akram Z, Safii SH, Vaithilingam RD, Baharuddin NA, Javed F, Vohra F. Efficacy of non-surgical periodontal therapy in the management of chronic periodontitis among obese and non-obese patients: a systematic review and meta-analysis. Clin Oral Investig. 2016;20(5):903–14.

Akram Z, Rahim ZH, Taiyeb-Ali TB, et al. Resistin as potential biomarker for chronic periodontitis: a systematic review and meta-analysis. Arch Oral Biol. 2017;73:311–20.

Baltacıoğlu E, Yuva P, Aydın G, et al. Lipid peroxidation levels and total oxidant/antioxidant status in serum and saliva from patients with chronic and aggressive periodontitis. Oxidative stress index: a new biomarker for periodontal disease? J Periodontol. 2014;85(10):1432–41.

Baňasová L, Kamodyová N, Janšáková K, et al. Salivary DNA and markers of oxidative stress in patients with chronic periodontitis. Clin Oral Investig. 2015;19(2):201–7.

Bertl K, Schoiber A, Haririan H, et al. Non-surgical periodontal therapy influences salivary melatonin levels. Clin Oral Investig. 2013;17(4):1219–25.

Bıyıkoğlu B, Buduneli N, Aksu K, et al. Periodontal therapy in chronic periodontitis lowers gingival crevicular fluid interleukin-1beta and DAS28 in rheumatoid arthritis patients. Rheumatol Int. 2013;33(10):2607–16.

Buduneli N, Bıyıkoğlu B, Sherrabeh S, Lappin DF. Saliva concentrations of RANKL and osteoprotegerin in smoker versus non-smoker chronic periodontitis patients. J Clin Periodontol. 2008; 35(10):846–52.

Buduneli N, Bıyıkoğlu B, İlgenli T, et al. Is obesity a possible modifier of periodontal disease as a chronic inflammatory process? A case-control study. J Periodontal Res. 2014;49(4):465–71.

Buhlin K, Hultin M, Noderyd O, et al. Risk factors for atherosclerosis in cases with severe periodontitis. J Clin Periodontol. 2009;36(7):541–9.

Costa PP, Trevisan GL, Macedo GO, et al. Salivary interleukin-6, matrix metalloproteinase-8, and osteoprotegerin in patients with periodontitis and diabetes. J Periodontol. 2010;81(3):384–91.

de Oliveira C, Watt R, Hamer M. Toothbrushing, inflammation, and risk of cardiovascular disease: results from Scottish Health Survey. BMJ. 2010;27(340):c2451.

Demmer RT, Trinquart L, Zuk A, et al. The influence of anti-infective periodontal treatment on C-reactive protein: a systematic review and meta-analysis of randomized controlled trials. PLoS One. 2013;8(10):e77441.

Dewhirst FE, Chen T, Izard J, et al. The human oral microbiome. J Bacteriol. 2010;192:5002–17.

Floriano PN, Christodoulides N, Miller CS, et al. Use of saliva-based nano-biochip tests for acute myocardial infarction at the point of care: a feasibility study. Clin Chem. 2009;55(8):1530–8.

Garlanda C, Maina V, Cotena A, Moalli F. The soluble pattern recognition receptor pentraxin-3 in innate immunity, inflammation and fertility. J Reprod Immunol. 2009;83:128–33.

Grassl N, Kulak NA, Pichler G, et al. Ultra-deep and quantitative saliva proteome reveals dynamics of the oral microbiome. Genome Med. 2016;8:44.

Gümüş P, Nizam N, Nalbantsoy A, Özçaka Ö, Buduneli N. Saliva and serum levels of pentraxin-3 and interleukin-1beta in generalized aggressive or chronic periodontitis. J Periodontol. 2014;85(3):e40–6.

Gümüş P, Özçaka Ö, Ceyhan-Öztürk B, Akcalı A, Lappin DF, Buduneli N. Evaluation of biochemical parameters and local and systemic levels of osteoactive and B-cell stimulatory factors in gestational diabetes in the presence or absence of gingivitis. J Periodontol. 2015;86(3):387–97.

Gümüş P, Kahraman-Çeneli S, Akcalı A, et al. Association of thalassemia major and gingival inflammation: a pilot study. Arch Oral Biol. 2016;64:80–4.

Gursoy UK, Könönen E, Pradhan-Palikhe P, et al. Salivary MMP-8, TIMP-1, and ICTP as markers of advanced periodontitis. J Clin Periodontol. 2010;37(6):487–93.

Gursoy UK, Könönen E, Pussinen PJ, et al. Use of host- and bacteria-derived salivary markers in detection of periodontitis: a cumulative approach. Dis Markers. 2011;30(6):299–305.

Hasuike A, Iguchi S, Suziki D, Kawano E, Sato S. Systematic review and assessment of systematic reviews examining the effect of periodontal treatment on glycemic control in patients with diabetes. Med Oral Patol Oral Cir Bucal. 2017;22(2):e167–76.

Heikkenen AM, Nwhator SO, Rathnayake N, Mantyla P, Vatanen P, Sorsa T. Pilot study on oral health status as assessed by an active matrix metalloproteinase-8 chairside mouthrinse test in adolescents. J Periodontol. 2016;87(1):36–40.

Jaedicke KM, Preshaw PM, Taylor JJ. Salivary cytokines as biomarkers of periodontal diseases. Periodontol 2000. 2016;70(1):164–83.

Kardeşler L, Buduneli N, Çetinkalp Ş, Kinane DF. Adipokines and inflammatory mediators after initial periodontal treatment in patients with type 2 diabetes and chronic periodontitis. J Periodontol. 2010;81(1):24–33.

Kinane DF, Chestnutt IG. Relationship of diabetes to periodontitis. Curr Opin Periodontol. 1997;4:29–34.

Kinney JS, Morelli T, Braun T, et al. Saliva/pathogen biomarker signatures and periodontal disease progression. J Dent Res. 2011;90(6):752–8.

Koga M, Kasayama S. Clinical impact of glycated albumin as another glycemic control marker. Endocr J. 2010;57:751–62.

Larsen T, Fiehn N-E. Dental biofilm infections–an update. APMIS. 2017;125:376–84.

Li S, Schmalz G, Schmidt J, Krause F, Haak R, Ziebolz D. Antimicrobial peptides as a possible interlink between periodontal diseases and its risk factors: a systematic review. J Periodontal Res. 2018;53(2):145–55.

Loos BG, Papantonopoulos G, Jepsen S, Laine ML. What is the contribution of genetics to periodontal risk? Dent Clin N Am. 2015;59(4):761–80.

Miller CS, King CP Jr, Langub MC, Kryscio RJ, Thomas MV. Salivary biomarkers of existing periodontal disease: a cross-sectional study. J Am Dent Assoc. 2006;137(3):322–9.

Miller CS, Foley JD 3rd, Floriano PN, et al. Utility of salivary biomarkers for demonstrating acute myocardial infarction. J Dent Res. 2014;93(7 Suppl):72S–9S.

Novakovic N, Todorovic T, Rakic M, et al. Salivary antioxidants as periodontal biomarkers in evaluation of tissue status and treatment outcome. J Periodontal Res. 2014;49(1):129–36.

Özçaka Ö, Ceyhan BÖ, Akcali A, Biçakci N, Lappin DF, Buduneli N. Is there an interaction between polycystic ovary syndrome and gingival inflammation? J Periodontol. 2012;83(12):1529–37.

Papapanou PN, Sanz M, Buduneli N, et al. Periodontitis: consensus report of workgroup 2 of the 2017 world workshop on the classification of periodontal and peri-implant diseases and conditions. J Clin Periodontol. 2018;45(Suppl 20):S162–70.

Paraskevas S, Huizinga JD, Loos BG. A systematic review and meta-analysis on C-reactive protein in relation to periodontitis. J Clin Periodontol. 2008;35(4):277–90.

Ramseier CA, Kinney JS, Herr AE, et al. Identification of pathogen and host-response markers correlated with periodontal disease. J Periodontol. 2009;80(3):436–46.

Sexton WM, Lin Y, Kryscio RJ, Dawson DR 3rd, Ebersole JL, Miller CS. Salivary biomarkers of periodontal disease in response to treatment. J Clin Periodontol. 2011;38(5):434–41.

Sivestre FJ, Silvestre-Rangil J, Bagan L, Bagan JV. Effect of nonsurgical periodontal treatment in patients with periodontitis and rheumatoid arthritis: a systematic review. Med Oral Patol Oral Cir Bucal. 2016;21(3):e349–54.

Tonetti MS, Greenwell H, Kornman KS. Staging and grading of periodontitis: framework and proposal of a new classification and case definition. J Clin Periodontol. 2018;45(Suppl 20):S149–61.

Tsuchida S, Satoh M, Takiwaki M, Nomura F. Current status of proteomic technologies for discovering and identifying gingival crevicular fluid biomarkers for periodontal disease. Int J Mol Sci. 2019;20:86.

Vidal F, Figueredo CM, Cordovil I, Fischer RG. Periodontal therapy reduces plasma levels of interleukin-6, C-reactive protein, and fibrinogen in patients with severe periodontitis and refractory arterial hypertension. J Periodontol. 2009;80(5):786–91.

Villa-Correa YA, Isaza-Guzmán DM, Tobón-Arroyave SI. Prognostic value of 8-hydroxy-2-deoxyguanosine and human neutrophil Elastase/α1-proteinase inhibitor complex as salivary biomarkers of oxidative stress in chronic periodontitis. J Periodontol. 2015;86(11):1260–7.

Yoshii S, Tsuboi S, Morita I, et al. Temporal association of elevated C-reactive protein and periodontal disease in men. J Periodontol. 2009;80(5):734–9.

Zhang L, Li X, Yan H, Huang L. Salivary matrix metalloproteinase (MMP-8) as a biomarker for periodontitis. A PRISMA-compliant systematic review and meta-analysis. Medicine. 2018;97(3):e9642.

9 Past, Present, and Future of Periodontics

9.1 Past

The consciousness about oral hygiene dates back to Sumerians 3000 BC, elaborately decorated gold toothpicks were found in the excavations at Ur in Mesopotamia. The Babylonians and Assyrians also seem to have suffered from periodontal problems, as a clay tablet of the period tells about treatment by gingival massage combined with herbal medications (Guerini 1909). Periodontal diseases were very common in Egyptians as evidenced in the embalmed bodies. The medical works of ancient India as well as ancient China devote a significant amount of space to oral and periodontal problems. In the ancient Greeks, Hippocrates of Cos, the father of modern medicine discussed the function and eruption of teeth and the aetiology of periodontal diseases. Among the Romans, 25 BC, diseases that affect the soft tissues of the mouth were mentioned. The Romans were very interested in oral hygiene and the use of toothbrush is mentioned in the writings of many Roman poets.

Periodontics flourished in central Europe, much later in the twentieth century, with two major centres of excellence: Vienna and Berlin. After World War II, the USA and Scandinavia took a leading role in basic and clinical periodontal research and the base of current periodontology was built. Most of the knowledge we have today about the nature of periodontal diseases is developed in mid-twentieth century.

Bernhard Gottlieb was in the Vienna Dental Group together with Orban, Sicher, Kronfeld, and Weinmann. During his era, diseases were classified as inflammatory, dystrophic, and neoplastic (Armitage 2002). He described for the first time marginal atrophy (gingivitis) and diffuse alveolar atrophy (periodontitis). Later on, two of his former students, Orban and Weinmann, renamed the disease as periodontosis. Gottlieb provided the basis for the interactions between the cells in the periodontium even in its primitive form, as cells talking to each other. Today we are aware of many signals or molecules that are derived from some cell types and act on some other cell types enabling the communication between cells.

In time due to the limitations of clinical diagnostic parameters, the search for biomarkers became popular in many different fields of medicine as well as dentistry. With the discovery of GCF, it was soon taken as a potential biofluid source for biomarkers of periodontal diseases.

Milestones in GCF research:

- Waerhaug (1966) focused on the anatomy of sulcus, its transformation into a pocket during the course of periodontitis.
- Brill (1962) laid the foundation for understanding the physiology of GCF formation, composition.
- Löe (1965) used GCF as an indicator of periodontal disease.

N. Buduneli, *Biomarkers in Periodontal Health and Disease*,
https://doi.org/10.1007/978-3-030-37317-7_9

- The first edition of the monograph "*The Crevicular Fluid*" by Cimasoni (1974) was published.

The followers do not know the difficulties that the pioneers faced while opening the pathway!

9.2 Present

Almost a century after Gottlieb's time, periodontal diseases are still a major global problem in large part due to the failure to implement what is known about their prevention. Moreover, the fact that they are still prevalent reflects a failure to understand the social determination of periodontal diseases. There is a failure on reliance on activities that dental practitioners can deliver to patients. It is also highly likely that there is a failure on advising people to adopt healthy behaviours and to avoid unhealthy ones.

At present, it is still early to depend on oral biomarkers alone in periodontal diagnosis, but they can be utilised to support the clinical parameters, which continue to be the most reliable diagnostic methods and also for monitoring disease progression.

You cannot always wait for the perfect time; sometimes you must dare to jump!

9.3 Future

One of the future challenges is to develop tests that evaluate the restoration of a health-associated homeostasis.

In the near future, the field of periodontal diagnostics will undergo major conceptual changes. One of the reasons behind this prediction is the intense research effort of medical and dental researchers to understand the impact of the human microbiome on health and disease. The microbiome consists of the diverse array of microbes that live on and in us throughout our lifespan. Together with bacteria, fungi, archaea, and viruses are all members of the human microbiome.

In the last 25 years, possible interactions or relationship between periodontal disease and numerous systemic diseases/conditions have been searched in cross-sectional or longitudinal studies as well as experimental animal models. Today, it is quite clear that there is a bidirectional relationship between periodontal diseases and diabetes. Uncontrolled or poorly controlled diabetes mellitus exacerbates the existent periodontal inflammation, increases the severity of periodontitis, and deteriorates the response to periodontal treatment. Similarly, severe periodontal inflammation deteriorates the metabolic control of diabetes, and successful periodontal treatment improves the metabolic control of the patient. A close relationship of periodontal diseases is suspected also with cardiovascular diseases, adverse pregnancy outcomes, rheumatoid arthritis, respiratory diseases, cognitive functions, etc.

There are also systemic conditions that share common pathological pathways with periodontal diseases and various systemic diseases. Obesity, metabolic syndrome, nutritional deficiencies are considered as examples for these.

Tobacco is one of the strongest addictive substances and its products affect periodontal health adversely, increase the extent and severity of periodontal diseases, and also worsen the response to periodontal treatment. The negative influence of tobacco products on the systemic health has been noticed earlier than that on oral health. In the context of harmful effects on systemic or oral health, active smoking is the worst and there is a dose-response relationship in many situations, but environmental smoking is now known to be harmful with significant effects also increasing with the frequency of severity of passive smoking. There have been national or governmental campaigns against tobacco products as it becomes more and more clear that tobacco gives tremendous harms to human health, is responsible for the vast majority of treatment costs, and is closely related with a vast majority of deaths all over the world. Tobacco industry has been producing new products to maintain their incomes and even worse they are targeting younger people to make them addicts. Waterpipe smoking rate has been increasing also in central Europe. Electronic cigarettes are advertised as being a remedy to stop smoking, but they are not! Dental professionals have a great responsibility to fight with tobacco products and they have a great power because dental treatment procedures usually require at least a few sessions, good communication is a critical factor for the long-term success of dental interventions, particularly periodontal treatment. Hence, dentists and dental hygienist inform their patients on the harmful effects of tobacco products and counsel them to stop smoking. Moreover, improving the society's consciousness about the harms of environmental smoking may help to widen non-smoking area and increase the number of never smokers.

Aesthetic concerns of the general population have been increasing particularly in the past 10–15 years. More and more people are getting concerned about their appearance and willing to look fit and young. Dental aesthetics has also gained a lot of interest. In fact, aesthetics should be taken as a whole and in terms of dental aesthetics white and pink aesthetics should be arm in arm. Tobacco products give striking harms by colouring the teeth and also leading to discolouration of gingiva, labial, and buccal mucosa. Dental professions can provide better aesthetics by counselling their patients to quit smoking!

Thus, in the future, dental professionals will be much more involved in the fight with tobacco! Counselling in cessation of smoking will be part of routine work for dental professionals. This is also a characteristic of the holistic treatment approach of today.

The studies bringing evidence for the common pathogenic pathways between periodontal diseases and various systemic diseases/conditions attract the interest from the medical and dental societies. A much closer communication and collaboration between dental professionals and physicians will provide significant improvements in the health state of the population.

Better clarifying the mechanisms of coupling of bone formation and bone resorption may lead to development of novel therapeutic approaches to guide cells for a complete regeneration. Future research will focus on stem cells and biologics combining cell-based therapies and controlled delivery of regulatory molecules using tissue-engineering techniques. When the complete picture behind bone formation and resorption is unravelled, it may be possible to achieve complete regeneration of lost periodontal structures. Understanding the cell-to-cell and cell-to-matrix interactions by proteomics and secretomics and using lab-on-a-chip technologies may bring out critical information for molecular therapies.

Possible modifying factors for regeneration of bone are epigenetic, age-related, environmental factors such as smoking, factors related with various drugs, and systemic diseases. Clarifying the mechanism of action will open up new pathways for successful periodontal treatment. Moreover, possible interactions between the oral microbiome and periodontal tissue cells, pathogenesis and healing remain to be better explained.

Macrophages have significant plasticity and play central roles in determining the tissue response to the microbial attacks from the dental biofilm. Various factors may stimulate macrophages to differentiate into either type-1 (M1) or type-2 (M2). M1 cells are more related with pro-inflammatory and M2 cells are related more with anti-inflammatory responses. A very recent study suggested that M2 phenotype is associated with decreased expression of RANKL and a reduced number of osteoclasts (Zhuang et al. 2019). Further clarification of the functions of M1 and M2 phenotypes will lead to the development of new treatment approaches aiming to modulate cytokines, chemokines, transcription factors, and micro-RNAs to influence a shift in the balance of M1 and M2 macrophages.

Advances in subject-based and site-based diagnostics will help to develop personalised/individually tailored treatment strategies. Such treatment approaches may improve the success of the treatment outcomes.

Goals to be achieved in the future:

1. Better definition of the roles and cross-talk of T-cell subsets in periodontitis,
2. Genome-wide studies better defining and correlating the transcriptomes and epigenomes of host cells in periodontal health and disease,
3. Clarifying whether dysbiosis is a cause or consequence of periodontal disease,
4. Definition of the molecular mechanisms by which periodontal bacteria inhibit antimicrobial or killing mechanisms without suppressing the overall inflammation,
5. Clarifying the mode of progression of periodontitis; whether it is linear or comprises episodes of active and quiescent periods,

6. Application of the progressing knowledge on pathogenesis to periodontal treatment for development of individually tailored therapeutic modalities.

Toll-like receptors (TLRs) seem to play a central role in the initiation and progression of periodontitis. However, further research is required to explain the effect of periodontopathogens on TLR expression, the interactions between bacteria, viruses, and TLRs. Moreover, developing simple and feasible ways to detect TLR levels in saliva, plasma, and GCF has a high potential in diagnosis and determination of prognosis in periodontal diseases (Song et al. 2017).

Combination tests focusing on certain cytokines, enzymes, and bacteria species may provide information on the cumulative risk and be more realistic as biomarker tests due to the complex and multifactorial nature of periodontal diseases. Within this context, IL-β and MMP-8 seem to be the most preferred mediators for determination of periodontal disease activity. MMP-8 deserves particular emphasis as it is contributing not only in initiation and progress of inflammation but also in healing. However, independent verification by extensive, prospective, large-scale, and multi-centre studies is warranted to have the basis for the clinical use of the currently available tests in the market. Molecular diagnostics in periodontal disease are to be encouraged, but not prematurely adopted.

In 1948 WHO defined health as "A state of complete physical, mental, and social wellbeing and not merely the absence of disease or infirmity". In 1993 Dolan defined the dental health as "A comfortable and functional dentition that allows individuals to continue their social life" (Dolan 1993). A more recent definition of oral health is as follows; "the ability to chew and eat the full range of foods native to the diet, to speak clearly, to have a socially acceptable smile and dentofacial profile, to be comfortable and free from pain and to have fresh breath" (Sheiham and Spencer 1997).

According to a more recent and comprehensive definition: "Oral health is multi-faceted and includes the ability to speak, smile, smell, taste, touch, chew, swallow, and convey a range of emotions through facial expressions with confidence and without pain, discomfort, and disease of the craniofacial complex". Further attributes include that it is a fundamental component of health and physical and mental wellbeing. It exists along a continuum influenced by the values and attitudes of individuals and communities; it reflects the physiologic, social, and psychological attributes that are essential to quality of life, it is influenced by the individual's changing experiences, perceptions, expectations, and ability to adapt to circumstances (Glick et al. 2016).

Things keep on changing. In fact, the only thing that does not change is that everything changes continuously in time. We all need to adapt to the current conditions and feel free to take steps forward rather than being strictly attached to our roots. The future of dentistry is bright with improvements in biomedical science, materials science, and close collaboration with physicians!

Chance favours only the prepared mind! Louis Pasteur

References

Armitage GC. Classifying periodontal diseases-a long-standing dilemma. Periodontol 2000. 2002;30:9–23.

Brill N. The gingival pocket fluid. Studies of its occurrence, composition and effect. Acta Odont Scand. 1962;20:(Suppl.32):1–115.

Cimasoni G. The crevicular fluid. Monogr Oral Sci. 1974;3:1–122.

Dolan T. Identification of appropriate outcomes for an aging population. Spec Care Dentist. 1993;13:35–9.

Glick M, Williams DM, Kleinman DV, Vujicic M, Watt RG, Weyant RJ. A new definition for oral health developed by the FDI world dental federation opens the door to a universal definition of oral health. JADA. 2016;147:915–7.

Guerini V. History of dentistry. Philadelphia, Lea & Febiger, 1909. NBBB.

Löe H. Physiology of the gingival pocket. Acad Rev Calif Acad Periodontol. 1965;13:6–14.

Sheiham A, Spencer J. Health needs assessment. In: Pine CM, editor. Community oral health. Oxford: Reed Educational and Professional Publishing Ltd; 1997. p. 39–54.

Song B, Zhang YL, Chen LJ, Zhou T, Huang WK, Zhou X, Shao LQ. The role of toll like receptors in periodontitis. Oral Dis. 2017;23:168–80.

Waerhaug J. Anatomy, physiology and pathology of the gingival pocket. Rev Belge Med Dent. 1966;21:9–15.

Zhuang Z, Yoshizawa-Smith S, Glowacki A, Maltos K, Pacheco C, Shehabeldin M, Sfeir C. Induction of M2 macrophages prevents bone loss in murine periodontitis models. J Dent Res. 2019;98:200–8.

MIX
Papier aus verantwortungsvollen Quellen
Paper from responsible sources
FSC® C105338

If you have any concerns about our products,
you can contact us on
ProductSafety@springernature.com

In case Publisher is established outside the EU,
the EU authorized representative is:
Springer Nature Customer Service Center GmbH
Europaplatz 3, 69115 Heidelberg, Germany

Printed by Libri Plureos GmbH
in Hamburg, Germany